An Atlas of
MYOCARDIAL INFARCTION

and related cardiovascular complications

THE ENCYCLOPEDIA OF VISUAL MEDICINE SERIES

An Atlas of
MYOCARDIAL INFARCTION
and related cardiovascular complications

Duncan S. Dymond

St. Bartholomew's Hospital
London, UK

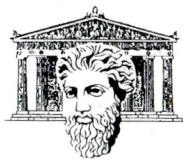

The Parthenon Publishing Group
International Publishers in Medicine, Science & Technology

NEW YORK   LONDON

British Library Cataloguing in Publication Data

Dymond, Duncan S.
   Atlas of Myocardial Infarction: And
   Related Cardiovascular Complications. –
   (Encyclopedia of Visual Medicine Series)
   I. Title II. Series
   616.1237
   ISBN 1-85070-505-4

Library of Congress Cataloging-in-Publication Data

Dymond, Duncan S.
   An atlas of myocardial infarction : and related cardiovascular
complications / Duncan S. Dymond.
     p.   cm. – (The Encyclopedia of visual medicine series)
   Includes bibliographical references and index.
   ISBN 1-85070-505-4
   1. Heart – Infarction – Atlases. I. Title. II. Series.
   [DNLM: 1. Myocardial Infarction – atlases.
   WG 17 D9966a 1994]
RC685.I6D95 1994
616.1' 237' 00222 – dc20
DNLM/DLC
for Library of Congress   94-21976
                             CIP

Published in the UK by
The Parthenon Publishing Group Limited
Casterton Hall, Carnforth
Lancs. LA6 2LA, England

Published in the USA by
The Parthenon Publishing Group Inc.
One Blue Hill Plaza
PO Box 1564, Pearl River
New York 10965, USA

Copyright © 1995 Parthenon Publishing Group Ltd.

Composition by Ryburn Publishing Services,
Keele University, Staffordshire, England
Printed and bound by Butler and Tanner Ltd,
Frome and London

Contents

The Encyclopedia of Visual Medicine Series

Titles currently planned in this series include:

An Atlas of Oncology
An Atlas of Hypertension
An Atlas of Common Diseases
An Atlas of Osteoporosis
An Atlas of Contraception
An Atlas of Endometriosis
An Atlas of Ultrasonography in Obstetrics and Gynecology
An Atlas of Practical Radiology
An Atlas of Psoriasis
An Atlas of Trauma Management
An Atlas of Lung Infections
An Atlas of Transvaginal Color Doppler
An Atlas of Infective Endocarditis
An Atlas of Rheumatology
An Atlas of Epilepsy
An Atlas of Differential Diagnosis in HIV Disease
An Atlas of Practical Dermatology
An Atlas of Laser Operative Laparoscopy and Hysteroscopy
An Atlas of Atherosclerosis
An Atlas of Eye Diseases
An Atlas of Cutaneous Growths
An Atlas of Myocardial Infarction

Foreword

The field of Medicine has made extraordinary advances in the past 20 years. Having said this, there is no discipline that has changed more radically than that of Cardiology. Dr Dymond has successfully travelled the course and has put together a well-illustrated atlas reflecting the current state of knowledge concerning myocardial infarction. Although ischemic heart disease remains the leading cause of death, there are some encouraging signs. Since 1985, when the mortality rate was 330 per 100000, this rate progressively fell to 292 per 100000 in 1990. The pathophysiology of acute myocardial infarction now concentrates on the importance of plaque rupture with subsequent formation of thrombus at the site of rupture. Dr Dymond amply illustrates this phenomenon with microscopic studies of coronary arteries. The section on diagnosis of acute myocardial infarction is laced with wisdom in that the frailties of patients denying their symptoms is highlighted. Once myocardial infarction occurs, a host of complications may follow. Dr Dymond chronicles and illustrates the full spectrum: cardiogenic shock, mitral regurgitation, myocardial rupture, ventricular aneurysms, pericarditis. Current concepts such as myocardial stunning and hibernation are discussed.

The text is a good summary of current knowledge of myocardial infarction, but the strength of this book rests with the illustrations. As our understanding of myocardial infarction has increased, so has the range of techniques with which we are able to study this disease. The Atlas is richly illustrated with electrocardiograms, angiograms, radionuclide scans, rest and stress echocardiograms, magnetic resonance images, holter monitors, angioscopy, and positron emission tomography images. It is in this section of the book that the reader marvels at the array of diagnostic tools that allows the physician to perform his magic. *An Atlas of Myocardial Infarction* is a strong statement of where we have been and where we currently are as we push the frontiers of science ahead of us. Dr Dymond has done a stellar job of chronicling this journey.

Lawrence S. Cohen, MD
Deputy Dean
Ebenezer K. Hunt Professor of Medicine
Yale University School of Medicine

Introduction

Apart from unheralded sudden cardiac death, myocardial infarction represents the most extreme expression of coronary artery disease. Myocardial infarction and sudden death are strongly interrelated. There is no doubt that the advent of Coronary Care Units, and the ability of paramedics to defibrillate patients unfortunate enough to suffer ventricular fibrillation as a consequence of myocardial infarction, have reduced the mortality due to this lethal arrhythmia. Until recently, cardiologists and physicians were relatively helpless to influence the amount of healthy heart muscle that was destined to become destroyed by the infarction process. The arrival of the thrombolytic era has changed that and it is now widely proven that thrombolytic therapy reduces in-hospital and long-term mortality from myocardial infarction by salvaging muscle from destruction. The way in which the myocardial infarction survivor is stratified according to future risk has become greatly refined in the last few years, and the imaging techniques available to delineate viable from non-viable myocardium are in a rapid phase of evolution. The prognostic tests in the post-infarct patient are by no means perfect, but it is possible to identify patients at high and low risk from future events. The complications of myocardial infarction, both electrical and mechanical, pose their own problems for management.

This volume is by no means a comprehensive textbook on myocardial infarction or electrocardiography. I have, however, attempted to put together a series of illustrations, ranging from pathology to interventional cardiology, that are both instructional and visually appealing and, whereas there may be certain omissions, I hope that the final volume will provide useful material for medical students, cardiologists in training and general physicians who have to cope with a large volume of myocardial infarction patients. I have included an extensive bibliography of further reading which is a reflection on how wide are the implications of acute myocardial infarction. I hope this further reading will prove of value.

Acknowledgements

In preparing this atlas, I would like to express gratitude to a number of friends and colleagues who have helped me to gather the material:

Professor R.W.F. Campbell, Department of Cardiology, Freeman Hospital, University of Newcastle-upon-Tyne, UK

Professor Michael Davies, St. George's Hospital Medical School, London, UK

Dr A. Lahiri, Department of Cardiology, Northwick Park Hospital, Harrow, Middlesex, UK

Dr Jamshid Maddahi, UCLA Clinical PET Center, Los Angeles, California, USA

Dr A.W. Nathan, Department of Cardiology, St. Bartholomew's Hospital, London, UK

Professor Michael Rees, Department of Radiology, North Staffordshire Hospital, Stoke-on-Trent, UK

Dr Richard Underwood, The Magnetic Resonance Unit, The Royal Brompton National Heart and Lung Hospitals, London, UK

Mark Monaghan, Cardiac Department, King's College Hospital, London, UK

I would also like to say a special thank you to Dr Richard Lim, former Research Registrar, Department of Cardiology, St. Bartholomew's Hospital, London, now Senior Registrar in Cardiology at Hull Royal Infirmary, and to Julie Dorrington at The National Slide Library, London for their help. Finally, I owe a special debt of gratitude to my friends and colleagues in The Department of Medical Photography at St. Bartholomew's Hospital for their infinite patience and cooperation during the preparation of this volume and to Sandra Brown for her superb secretarial assistance.

Section 1   A Review of Myocardial Infarction

Introduction and epidemiology

In 1789 Benjamin Franklin wrote, in a letter to Jean Baptiste Leroy, 'but in this world nothing can be said to be certain, except death and taxes'. As shown in Table 1, ischemic heart disease has ranked number one for two decades as the leading cause of both male and female deaths in the United Kingdom, and the majority of those deaths are due to acute myocardial infarction. Table 2 shown that ischemic heart disease is the single most common *identifiable* cause of death, with 292 deaths per 100 000 of the population in 1990. Deaths from coronary heart disease are four times more common than deaths due to lung cancer. The mortality rate seemed to reach a peak in 1985 and has fallen slowly but steadily since that time, from 330 per 100 000 in 1985 to 292 per 100 000 in 1990. These unwelcome statistics span the entire age range and Tables 3 and 4 show the male and female deaths, respectively per 100 000 of the population, both for all ages and for various individual age brackets. Even in women between the ages of 45 and 64, ischemic heart disease is a commoner cause of fatality than breast cancer. Looking at it another way, Table 5 shows the years (in thousands) of life lost due to premature deaths, i.e. under the age of 64, in England and Wales for various diseases. Once again, ischemic heart disease is the most common single cause of loss of life and causes nearly four times as many years of life to be lost as cerebrovascular disease and only slightly less than all accidental deaths. Table 6 shows that when one examines the percentage of distribution of years lost due to male deaths under the age of 64, ischemic heart disease remained constantly higher than those due to all other diseases at 82%.

Table 1   Ranking of leading causes of deaths (male and female), UK. Source: Annual Abstract of Statistics

	1970	1980	1985	1986	1987	1988	1989	1990
Ischemic heart disease	1	1	1	1	1	1	1	1
Cerebrovascular disease	2	2	2	2	2	2	2	2
Cancer of lung/trachea/bronchus	4	4	3	3	3	3	3	3
Pneumonia	3	3	4	4	4	4	4	4
Diseases of pulmonary circulation*	6	5	5	5	5	5	5	5
Cancer of breast	8	7	7	6	6	6	6	6
Cancer of stomach	7	8	8	8	7	7	7	7

* Including other forms of heart disease

Table 2   Leading causes of deaths (male and female) as per 100 000 population, UK. Source: Annual Abstract of Statistics

	1970	1980	1985	1986	1987	1988	1989	1990
Ischemic heart disease	290	314	330	320	313	308	303	292
Cerebrovascular disease	165	147	148	145	140	137	136	132
Cancer of lung/trachea/bronchus	62	71	72	71	71	70	69	68
Pneumonia	84	104	59	59	52	56	62	53
Diseases of pulmonary circulation*	57	69	47	44	42	42	43	39
Cancer of breast	22	24	27	27	27	27	28	27
Cancer of stomach	26	22	20	19	19	19	18	17
Diabetes mellitus	10	10	14	15	14	15	15	16
Bronchitis, emphysema and asthma	59	38	27	23	19	17	17	14
Motor vehicle accidents	14	12	10	10	10	9	10	10
Gastric/duodenal ulcer	8	9	10	9	8	8	9	9
Nephritis, nephrotic syndrome	5	9	10	9	9	9	9	8
Leukemia	6	7	7	7	7	7	7	7
Hypertensive disease	20	11	9	8	7	7	7	6
Cancer of uterus	8	7	7	7	7	7	6	6
Chronic liver disease and cirrhosis	3	5	5	5	6	6	6	6
Chronic rheumatic heart disease	15	6	6	5	5	5	5	4

* Including other forms of heart disease

It seems certain that the most common cause of sudden death in the adult population is coronary artery disease. Sudden death has been reported to be the first clinical manifestation of acute myocardial infarction in between 20 and 25% of all cases. Of more than 500 000 coronary deaths per year, fully 60% are unheralded. Additionally, the fraction of coronary deaths occurring suddenly appears to be higher in young adults than in the older population. Sudden unexpected unheralded death still poses one of the greatest medical problems to cardiologists and physicians in the Western world. Although acute myocardial infarction and sudden death are inexorably linked, and although 40–60% of fatalities from acute myocardial

Table 3   Male deaths per 100 000 population (age specific), England and Wales, 1990. Source: OPCS

		Age (years)				
	All ages	< 24	25–44	45–64	65–74	> 75
Ischemic heart disease	330	0	19	325	1318	2959
Cerebrovascular disease	101	1	4	48	304	1307
Cancer of lung/trachea/bronchus	96	0	3	105	455	707
Pneumonia	39	1	3	10	61	622
Cancer of prostate	33	0	0	12	117	414
Diseases of pulmonary circulation*	31	1	4	20	75	376
Bronchitis, emphysema and asthma	22	1	1	13	86	239
Cancer of colon	22	0	1	22	88	189
Cancer of stomach	21	0	1	21	92	179
Diabetes mellitus	14	0	1	9	46	159

* Including other forms of heart disease

Table 4   Female deaths per 100 000 population (age specific), England and Wales, 1990. Source: OPSC

	All ages	< 24	25–44	45–64	65–74	> 75
			Age (years)			
Ischemic heart disease	256	0	3	97	571	2000
Cerebrovascular disease	161	0	4	35	232	1439
Pneumonia	66	1	1	6	43	664
Cancer of breast	53	0	12	79	135	218
Diseases of pulmonary circulation*	47	1	1	10	50	440
Cancer of lung/trachea/bronchus	41	0	2	47	164	165
Cancer of colon	24	0	2	18	64	151
Diabetes mellitus	17	0	1	8	37	130
Bronchitis, emphysema and asthma	13	1	1	10	35	80
Cancer of stomach	13	0	1	7	33	94

* Including other forms of heart disease

infarction may occur before arrival at a medical facility, there are still vast numbers of patients who survive their infarction and in whom in-hospital mortality and long-term mortality can be reduced by careful monitoring and early treatment of arrhythmias, and by prompt treatment with thrombolytic therapy or, in some cases, direct angioplasty.

The way in which the so-called 'uncomplicated infarct' is handled has changed in the last 15 years and the assessment of prognosis has become as important as the treatment of the acute event itself. There would be little point in carrying out a detailed assessment of prognosis and likelihood of future infarction or late death unless one could modify that prognosis with a suitable intervention. Not every procedure that is carried out has been the subject of rigorous randomized trials, but, with the passage of each year, more data become available on interventions which seem to prolong life in the postinfarct patient.

Table 5   Years of life lost* due to premature deaths (male and female), England and Wales. Source: OPCS

	1980	1982	1984	1986	1988	1989	1990
All malignant neoplasms	431	410	420	392	393	384	375
Circulatory diseases	447	405	377	345	312	297	289
ischemic heart disease	289	263	252	230	206	192	187
cerebrovascular disease	76	70	64	59	54	51	50
All accidental deaths	240	231	215	202	189	196	205
Suicide	70	71	72	72	81	73	81
Respiratory system	135	121	81	74	73	70	66

* Years (in thousands) of life lost relate to ages 15–64

Table 6   Percentage distribution of years lost*due to male deaths. Source: OPCS

	1980	1982	1984	1986	1988	1989	1990
All malignant neoplasms	49%	49%	49%	47%	48%	48%	48%
Circulatory diseases	73%	73%	74%	75%	74%	74%	74%
ischemic heart disease	82%	82%	82%	82%	82%	82%	82%
cerebrovascular disease	54%	53%	54%	56%	53%	55%	54%
All accidental deaths	77%	76%	77%	76%	78%	78%	78%
Suicide	68%	73%	75%	77%	79%	81%	81%
Respiratory system	59%	60%	59%	61%	58%	60%	60%

* Years of life lost relate to ages 15–64

Risk factors for coronary disease

Postmortem studies of arteries from different racial groups around the world, and in the young as well as the old, have shown that atherosclerosis begins early in life with fatty streaks being obvious in the thoracic and abdominal aortas as early as the age of 16. However, there are large differences world-wide in the incidence and mortality rates from coronary heart disease, and the relationship between the presence of fatty streaks and clinical arterial disease is a continuing subject of debate. Raised or obstructive lesions correspond well with the ranking of mortality due to atherosclerotic heart disease. Severe atherosclerosis may be primarily due to environmental conditions and geography, although certain racial groups do seem to show a higher than normal incidence of clinical coronary disease at younger ages. Smoking, diabetes, hypertension and a family history are all strongly associated with coronary heart disease. It is sometimes difficult to separate family history from other self-inflicted risk factors such as smoking. For example, if five brothers who die of coronary disease all smoked, does this mean that the one non-smoking brother is at equal risk of coronary heart disease? Why is it that some people can smoke 60 cigarettes a day and not develop heart disease whereas others will? These questions remain largely unanswered. More recently, a raised blood cholesterol level, and particularly a raised low density lipoprotein (LDL) level with a low high density lipoprotein (HDL) level, would seem to have been proven to be related to coronary heart disease. It is now becoming more accepted that there is a strong relationship between a raised triglyceride level and coronary disease. Other factors such as obesity are more difficult to prove because of the high incidence of diabetes and raised triglycerides among obese people. The fact that myocardial infarction, rare (although not unknown) in premenopausal women suggests that estrogens may confer a protective effect on the vascular endothelium. This has been the basis for the administration of hormone replacement therapy (HRT) to postmenopausal women, since HRT may protect against coronary disease as well as against other conditions such as osteoporosis. Clearly, the epidemiological approach to the true causes of coronary disease and the relevance of the risk factors in converting a benign process into a potentially lethal one will be the subject of much ongoing research.

Acute myocardial infarction and plaque rupture

Recent studies have clarified the interaction between coronary atheroma and thrombus formation in patients with a variety of ischemic syndromes, including crescendo angina and acute myocardial infarction. The build-up of a significant plaque may take decades but acute thrombus formation may take place in a matter of minutes. Postmortem studies have shown that coronary thrombosis in fatal cases of acute myocardial infarction is nearly always related to plaque rupture. This leads to free communication between blood flowing through the coronary artery and the lipid-rich center of the plaque. Blood from the lumen of the coronary artery dissects into the plaque, producing a large intraluminal thrombus which is platelet-rich. This thrombus may propagate within the lumen, even into segments that do not have any actual disease in them. Plaque rupture with thrombus formation appears to be a common pathophysiological event in patients who present with unstable angina, patients who survive acute myocardial infarction, or patients with sudden death. A totally occlusive thrombus is more likely to be associated with a myocardial infarction and non-occlusive thrombus with crescendo angina or perhaps a smaller infarction. Angioscopic studies have recently demonstrated thrombus associated with these events in live patients.

Although plaque rupture appears to be an unpredictable event, recent studies have shown that there is a circadian variation in the frequency of onset of myocardial infarction. There is a peak between 06.00 and noon, and a secondary peak late in the evening, even in patients who are already on β-blockers.

The Framingham study demonstrated a peak incidence of sudden death between 09.00 and 11.00 (in the morning) and implied a possible relationship of physical and mental activity to plaque rupture and fatal arrhythmias.

Others have suggested an important role for the vasa vasorum in the pathogenesis of intramural hemorrhage. The walls of an atherosclerotic artery are rich in capillary vessels of the vasa vasorum. Surges in blood pressure in the morning may make these fragile neovascular structures more prone to rupture. The MILIS study demonstrated that 48% of their study population had undergone physical exertion or suffered an emotional upset immediately prior to the onset of an acute myocardial infarction. Patients who undergo a plaque fissure and who do not present with unstable angina, acute myocardial infarction or sudden death are usually left with an atherosclerotic plaque which is far larger than before and the thrombus undergoes organization inside the plaque. It is possible that such episodic plaque enlargement is an important factor in the development of angina pectoris at a later stage.

The demonstration that up to 80% of patients with acute myocardial infarction have coronary thrombosis has led to the wide use of thrombolytic therapy in order to dissolve the clot and restore antegrade flow down the infarct-related artery. As will be discussed later, this has been one of the major achievements of modern cardiology and has led to significant reductions in mortality.

Diagnosis of acute myocardial infarction

By far the most important feature is the history. It is a human frailty that patients who have been experiencing cardiac chest pain for some days may fail to recognize it as cardiac and be treated for 'indigestion'. The author knows at least half a dozen excellent general practitioners who have been treating themselves for indigestion, whereas a similar pain in a patient would have promoted instant referral to hospital with a presumptive diagnosis of cardiac pain. Patients may often perceive the symptoms not as pain but as chest tightness and the sensation in the arms may be described as a heaviness or leadenness, rather than pain. Some patients present with shortness of breath rather than pain or tightness, but an associated history of sweating, pain in the jaw or teeth and shortness of breath are of value. Most cardiologists would be fairly dogmatic in teaching that any patient with suspected cardiac pain, even if it is somewhat atypical, should be admitted to hospital. The presence of a normal electrocardiogram upon presentation does not rule out unstable angina or a myocardial infarction, and patients should not be discharged from a medical facility on the basis of a normal electrocardiogram (ECG) if the history is suspicious. It is important to ascertain at the time of presentation whether there are any risk factors for coronary artery disease as, clearly, atypical symptoms in a smoking, hypertensive diabetic with a bad family history will tilt the balance of probabilities towards a cardiac diagnosis whatever the ECG may show. The electrocardiographic criteria for the diagnosis of acute myocardial infarction are well described in many textbooks and some examples are used as illustrations in this atlas. The purpose of the electrocardiogram should to be to confirm what one suspects clinically, and one might even go a stage further and state that the ECG should only be used to determine whether a patient is eligible for immediate thrombolytic therapy or not. As thrombolytic therapy has not been shown to reduce mortality in patients with crescendo angina, then the presence of a normal ECG, or ST segment depression rather than elevation, may lead the clinician to prescribe intravenous nitrates and heparin rather than streptokinase or tissue plasminogen activator. The ECG may be very unhelpful if it shows complete left bundle branch block or if there is a paced rhythm. Other confusing pictures may be due to pericarditis, although the pattern of ST segment elevation is usually different, or in patients with high take-off ST segments which are a normal variant in some races.

Until the thrombolytic era, it was generally accepted that the development of Q waves meant a fixed scar replacing viable myocardium at the site of the infarction. The terms 'transmural infarction' for a Q wave infarct and 'subendocardial' for an infarct associated with T wave changes only are probably best avoided, as not all Q wave infarcts are in fact transmural. In the thrombolytic era, it has now become apparent that one may have well-developed Q waves on the electrocardiogram without the development of fixed scar tissue. The assessment of left ventricular function by two-dimensional echocardiography, radionuclide angiography or contrast angiography may often show well preserved contraction at the site of electrocardiographic Q waves. Prompt thrombolytic therapy may well convert what was destined to be a Q wave myocardial infarction into a non-Q wave infarction

The cardiac enzyme profile associated with myocardial infarction is well known. Creatine phosphokinase is the first enzyme to be elevated when myocardial cell membrane integrity is lost. It has often been felt that the peak creatine phosphokinase is a reflection of the size of the infarction, although in the thrombolytic era an early high peak of creatine phosphokinase may reflect successful thrombolysis and reperfusion, and increase the amount of creatine phosphokinase in the blood without implying a massive infarction.

Certain radiopharmaceuticals have been shown to accumulate inside freshly infarcted tissue. In the 1970s technetium-99m stannous pyrophosphate was shown to be able to identify and localize the site of infarction accurately, although the exact mechanism of its uptake remained unclear. Recently, ^{111}In-labelled anti-myosin, a monoclonal antibody to cardiac muscle protein, has also been shown to accumulate in acutely infarcted tissue, and examples of images using both these agents are shown in this atlas. In everyday clinical practice, it is rare to need such positive myocardial scintigraphy to make the diagnosis of acute myocardial infarction, but, in cases where the electrocardiogram and cardiac enzymes are unhelpful or equivocal, these techniques do have a role to play. It is of interest that, in patients with unstable angina whose enzymes remain normal, the scintigrams may well show islands of necrotic tissue, confirming that the conditions of unstable angina and myocardial infarction are in fact different manifestations of the same pathophysiological process.

Reciprocal ST segment depression

It is not at all uncommon, in patients with an inferior myocardial infarction with ST segment elevation in the inferior leads, to see ST segment depression in the precordial leads. Similarly, patients with anterior myocardial infarction may show ST segment depression in the inferior leads. These have been known as reciprocal changes and their significance has been the subject of much debate. It has been suggested that patients with inferior myocardial infarction who manifest ST segment depression anteriorly have a higher incidence of a separate stenosis in the left anterior descending artery than patients who do not have ST segment depression, and hence the pattern has been used to try and predict multi-vessel coronary disease. However, a dominant right coronary artery may well provide some blood supply to the lower part of the interventricular septum and it is, therefore, not surprising that published studies have failed to demonstrate a uniform pattern of coronary disease in patients with and without the phenomenon of reciprocal ST segment changes. Because of individual variations in coronary anatomy, it is unwise to assume one can relate changes in a particular area of myocardium to any particular coronary artery and reciprocal ST segment changes may not always mean a separate lesion in an artery other than the infarct-related vessel.

Arrhythmias

The most lethal arrhythmia complicating acute myocardial infarction is ventricular fibrillation and this may account for a large proportion of the sudden deaths. Ventricular fibrillation occurs in 10–15% of patients suffering an acute myocardial infarction. There is no doubt that the broadening of education of the general public in the administration of cardiopulmonary resuscitation, together with the increased availability of paramedics armed with defibrillators and skilled in intubation, has saved numerous lives. The proliferation of coronary care units and of nursing staff trained in coronary care has enabled prompt anti-arrhythmic therapy to be instituted once the patient gets to hospital. Primary ventricular fibrillation complicating the acute myocardial infarction is eminently treatable and, as long as oxygenation and cardiac massage are carried out if a defibrillator is not immediately available, then there is no reason why a satisfactory outcome should not be obtained. There has been some debate about the significance of early ventricular fibrillation as an independent prognostic indicator in survivors of acute myocardial infarction. Some have suggested that it is associated with a poorer in-hospital prognosis, although others have disagreed. It is generally accepted, however, that primary ventricular fibrillation does not have a major adverse effect on long-term outcome after hospital discharge. Secondary ventricular fibrillation, i.e. ventricular fibrillation remote from the actual infarction, has also been suggested by some to be a poor prognostic sign with in some cases up to a 50–60% in-hospital mortality. Late ventricular fibrillation is often associated with larger infarcts, and a higher incidence of heart failure and hypotension.

More recent studies have suggested that secondary ventricular fibrillation *per se* is not an independent poor prognostic indicator but that heart failure, hypotension or the presence of a gallop rhythm are more likely to indicate a poor prognosis as they are all markers of poor left ventricular function.

Bradycardias of various kinds are common complications of inferior or posterior myocardial infarction. The sinus node artery arises from the right coronary artery, and sinus bradycardia, sinus pauses or even prolonged sinus arrest are common features of inferior myocardial infarction. The prognosis from this is very good, however, but although patients who do not respond to intravenous atropine may require temporary pacing, permanent pacing is rarely required. The atrioventricular node has a dual blood supply from the right coronary artery and the circumflex, and temporary atrioventricular block is again a common feature of inferior myocardial infarction. Often, the escape rhythm is junctional at quite a respectable rate and temporary pacing is only needed if the escape focus is unreliable or if the patient is hypotensive, oliguric or has symptoms of dizziness associated with a slow heart rate. Most patients will return to sinus rhythm, although it may take up to 3 weeks to do so. Second-degree heart block of the Wenckebach type rarely requires temporary pacing. Whereas heart block in inferior myocardial infarction can be associated with only minor myocardial damage, this is not the case for anterior infarction. If the left anterior descending branch occludes and the interventricular septum is damaged, then the conduction tissues localized in the septum may be damaged permanently. This may lead to right bundle branch block, right bundle branch block with left anterior or left posterior hemiblock, left bundle branch block, or second-degree heart block of the Mobitz II variety.

Complete heart block after an anterior myocardial infarction will require permanent pacing. The need for permanent pacing in a patient with an anterior myocardial infarction and bifascicular block, with or without a prolongation of the PR interval, has been the subject of much debate.

Right ventricular infarction

It is only relatively recently that right ventricular infarction has been recognized as an important clinical entity. In a postmortem study of 2000 hearts, right ventricular infarction was demonstrated in just under 14%, mainly as an extension from the left ventricle, but in 2.4% infarction was confined entirely to the right ventricle. Right ventricular involvement is much more common in inferior myocardial infarction than in anterior infarction, occurring with an incidence reported as between 19% and 51%. It is also claimed to be a strong indicator of possible mortality in patients with an inferior myocardial infarction. Scintigraphic studies have suggested that right ventricular function may be acutely depressed in patients with an inferior myocardial infarction but that it does tend to return to normal after a while. It is very important to recognize right ventricular infarction clinically. A raised right ventricular end-diastolic pressure will cause a raised right atrial pressure and a rise in the patient's jugular venous pressure. This can be erroneously taken to indicate heart failure, and diuretics may be inappropriately given. If diuretics lower the right ventricular filling pressure too low, then the patient may become hypotensive with a poor cardiac output and oliguria. A raised jugular venous pulse in the absence of evidence of pulmonary venous congestion on chest X-ray should alert the clinician to the possibility of right ventricular infarction and, paradoxically, many of these patients may require fluid in order to increase the driving pressure to the right ventricle rather than diuretics. Right atrial pressure in right ventricular infarction will be higher than the pulmonary capillary wedge pressure. That is not to say that patients with extensive anterior myocardial infarction and left ventricular dysfunction will not suffer right ventricular dysfunction secondarily. The clinical skill lies in the recognition of isolated right ventricular infarction as the primary problem.

Treatment and prognosis

Thrombolysis

Several large studies have now shown beyond any reasonable doubt that the prompt administration of thrombolytic therapy reduces in-hospital mortality and out of hospital mortality rates. Studies such as GISSI, ISIS-2, AIMS, and ASSET have all shown statistically improved survival with successful thrombolytic therapy. Thus, major inroads have been made upon the loss of functioning myocardium which contributes so much to morbidity and mortality after myocardial infarction. The recently published ISIS-3 study showed no real differences between streptokinase and tissue plasminogen activator, although the latter was associated with a slightly higher incidence of hemorrhagic strokes. The key to successful thrombolysis is the recognition of electrocardiographic patterns which make a patient eligible for thrombolysis, and to minimize so-called 'pain to needle time', as it has been well shown that the earlier the thrombolytic therapy can be administered, the greater the benefit to the patient. Studies are also being conducted on the feasibility of prehospital thrombolytic therapy being administered in the patient's office or home, rather than waiting until the patient arrives at hospital. Although there are insufficient studies to suggest this confers a definite additional benefit, the idea is an attractive one, although the logistics of carrying this out will vary from city to city and country to country. The need for heparin post-thrombolysis has also been the subject of some argument. Current wisdom seems to indicate that subcutaneous heparin will suffice after streptokinase, but intravenous heparin is necessary after tissue plasminogen activator. The other important factor in the administration of thrombolysis is to make sure that one adheres to the adage 'primum non nocere'. In other words, the drug must not make the patient worse. One must adhere strictly to exclusion critena so that patients with proliferative retinopathy are not put at risk of blindness and patients with a history of a recent hemorrhagic stroke or recent major surgery are not put at risk of major bleeding complications. There has been a tendency to withhold thrombolytic therapy in the elderly, although studies have shown that they benefit just as much as the younger population from restoration of arterial patency. Patients may often experience reperfusion arrhythmias during lytic therapy. Usually this is a benign phenomenon and may produce a few episodes of non-sustained ventricular tachycardia, but, more rarely, ventricular fibrillation requiring the administration of a direct current countershock may be necessary. Blood pressure must be closely monitored during streptokinase administration as allergic reactions are not all that uncommon and the infusion should be stopped if such a reaction occurs. Many individuals cover the administration of streptokinase with some intravenous hydrocortisone, although this is by no means a universal practice.

Once the patient has recovered from the infarct, a largely unresolved question is 'What should one do next'? Opinions and philosophies differ widely in the cardiological community. Some believe that every patient who has had thrombolytic therapy should have a coronary angiogram, and, if there is a tight residual stenosis, this should be treated by angioplasty, or, if there is multi-vessel disease, the patient should undergo coronary bypass surgery without any further ado. Others feel that only patients who demonstrate recurrent symptoms or who have evidence of inducible ischemia on exercise stress testing or with radionuclide stress testing should undergo invasive examination with a view to intervention. The problem has arisen because it is very difficult to predict which patients will reocclude and hence reinfarct, and which patients will come back with future cardiac events remote from their infarct. One trial that has been performed to date was the TAMI trial, published in 1987, which showed that an immediate angioplasty to a vessel which had been treated by thrombolysis produced a worse outcome than delaying the investigation for approximately 10–14 days. Several studies have tried to examine which criteria can predict reocclusion but results have differed. A recently published study (the APRICOT study) did suggest that, where there was a high-grade stenosis of more than 90%, there was a higher risk of reocclusion (42% compared to only a 23% risk of reocclusion in stenoses of less than 90%). Not all published studies would support this, however, and the dilemma continues. It is certainly tempting for interventional cardiologists to perform an angioplasty on a vessel that demonstrates a tight stenosis after thrombolysis. No one knows whether this is really the right thing to do in the absence of symptoms or of significant inducible ischemia. More randomized trials are required in large numbers of patients.

Primary angioplasty

Primary angioplasty refers to the practice of direct recanalization of an infarct-related vessel with angioplasty without prior thrombolysis. The studies that have been published suggest that the treatment is successful and, by definition, the residual stenosis after direct angioplasty is less than with thrombolysis alone. The mortality rates are acceptably low but the main problem in the wide acceptance of this technique is the logistic one. Even in the United States not every institution with a cardiac catheter laboratory can offer a 24-hour service for direct angioplasty for infarct patients. Most interventional cardiologists would agree that, where thrombolysis is contraindicated, direct angioplasty should be carried out if at all possible to restore vessel patency, and this can be very rewarding.

Primary angioplasty has also been carried out in patients who have had previous coronary bypass surgery who present with myocardial infarction. Unfortunately, if the angioplasty is carried out directly into the vein graft rather than the native vessel, the restenosis rate may be as high as 71%. Perhaps stent implantation into the graft will solve this problem.

β-blockers postinfarction

Several studies have shown that β-blockers are beneficial as a secondary prevention measure in reducing reinfarction and mortality rates after an uncomplicated myocardial infarction. There appears to be no benefit in giving β-blockers immediately, but starting them in the convalescent phase has reduced the 3-year mortality compared to patients not treated in this manner. The BetaBlocker Heart Attack Trial experience randomized nearly 4000 patients to treat them with either propranolol or placebo, and found a 20% reduction in mortality in the propranolol group. This was in spite of the 17% rise in triglyceride levels and a 6% rise in low density lipoprotein levels in the propranolol-treated group.

Exercise testing and isotope testing postinfarction and their relation to prognosis

In the last decade, a host of studies have been published examining the prognostic value of exercise testing soon after myocardial infarction, in an attempt to predict multivessel coronary disease, or future cardiac events such as unstable angina, reinfarction or death. Exercise testing before the patient leaves hospital is usually carried out using a submaximal protocol, where the endpoint is a 50% increase in the patient's heart rate over resting levels. An abnormal exercise test before discharge, whether it be chest pain on the treadmill, ST segment changes in a site remote from the infarction, arrhythmias or an abnormal blood pressure response, may provoke a predischarge coronary angiogram and revascularization if necessary. It is now quite common, if a patient has a normal predischarge exercise test, to repeat it at 6 weeks using a maximal protocol. Thallium-201 scanning or, more recently, scanning with one of the technetium-99m perfusion scanning agents such as MIBI has also proved useful in identifying ischemia remote from the site of the infarction. Exercise radionuclide ventriculography, where left ventricular function is assessed at rest and at peak exercise, has also been used successfully in identifying remote ischemia, and is helpful in determining which patients should undergo invasive investigation.

The role of the exercise test after myocardial infarction has required some rethinking in the thrombolytic era. The exercise test has not proved useful in predicting which patients will reocclude the lysed vessel, although clearly patients with an abnormal exercise test and widespread exercise-induced ischemia will have a strong probability of having an angiogram with a view to revascularization. A negative treadmill test after thrombolysis, however, does not necessarily imply a good prognosis, in terms of reocclusion.

Left ventricular function

Despite all the advances that have been made in the last 10–15 years in terms of risk stratification, poor left ventricular function remains the overwhelming factor which dictates an adverse prognosis in survivors of acute myocardial infarction. The simple measurement of left ventricular ejection fraction, be it by echocardiography or radionuclide ventriculography, still remains the most powerful predictor of prognosis. In some studies, patients with an ejection fraction of less than 20% have a 50% 1-year mortality, whereas patients with an ejection fraction greater than 50% have a 1-year mortality of only 1–2%. Patients with poor left ventricular function are more prone to severe and life-threatening ventricular arrhythmias, and to repeated hospital admissions for congestive cardiac failure. They are often on large amounts of medications which produce side-effects, and they suffer the consequences of a low cardiac output by having a high risk of developing renal impairment, for example.

Life-threatening arrhythmias are the most dramatic expression of poor left ventricular function. Patients who present with ventricular tachycardia, which may degenerate into ventricular fibrillation, are an immense management problem. The scope for administering antiarrhythmic drugs is limited in such patients because of the negative inotropic effects of many of the drugs, which may precipitate or worsen congestive cardiac failure. In addition, many of the antiarrhythmic drugs, especially those in the Class I group, have a pro-arrhythmic effect in patients with poor left ventricular function. In particular, flecainide may well be contraindicated in such patients. β-Blockers may be poorly

tolerated in patients with depressed left ventricular function. Amiodarone is the antiarrhythmic of choice for suppressing arrhythmias in patients with poor left ventricular function, and in many cases may be successful in preventing or reducing the frequency of attacks of ventricular arrhythmias. It is sometimes used in combination with a drug such as mexiletine. Electrophysiological studies have been widely used to test the inducibility of ventricular arrhythmias using medications, but sometimes arrhythmias that occur spontaneously cannot be induced in the laboratory, and it is hard to know exactly whether a patient is safe on a medication. This has led to the development and use of the automatic implantable cardioverter defibrillator (AICD). This device recognizes ventricular tachycardia or ventricular fibrillation and defibrillates the patient out of hospital. Extensive experience is being gained with this device and, hopefully, many lives will be saved.

An alternative approach to the use of the defibrillator is a surgical one, whereby the scarred endocardium responsible for the ventricular arrhythmia is resected surgically or even cryoablated at operation. The success of these procedures is variable, and, of course, patients with very poor left ventricular function will have an increased mortality rate undergoing such surgery. Cardiac transplantation may be considered in the younger patient with malignant arrhythmias as an alternative to the use of the defibrillator.

Infarct expansion and cardiac dilatation

Progressive left ventricular dilatation has been shown to occur as a function of size and age of a myocardial infarction. During the early postinfarction phase, the left ventricular end-diastolic volume increases as a consequence of the expansion of the infarct and an increase in filling pressure. The left ventricle may continue to dilate as a result of the process of remodelling of the viable myocardium. In infarcts of sufficient size, ventricular volume may go on increasing, leading to further deterioration in ventricular performance. It has been shown in the rat model that the long-term administration of angiotensin converting enzyme (ACE) inhibitors attenuates this gradual left ventricular enlargement. Recently, clinical studies have confirmed that ACE inhibitors may prevent ventricular enlargement in humans. In humans, two studies have shown that patients who are prescribed captopril after a

Q wave myocardial infarction without overt heart failure have a smaller increase in left ventricular volume than in patients given placebo. It, therefore, seems possible that ACE inhibitors may alter their remodelling process and improve long-term prognosis. The CONSENSUS trial showed an improved survival in patients with symptomatic left ventricular failure and ACE inhibitors are now used routinely in these patients.

Other complications of myocardial infarction

Apart from malignant ventricular arrhythmias and progressive left ventricular dilatation and heart failure, other more specific complications require some comment.

Cardiogenic shock

Cardiogenic shock is a condition characterized by hypotension (< 90 mmHg systolic), oliguria (< 30 ml urine/hour), sweating and sometimes mental confusion. When cardiogenic shock is due to overwhelming loss of functioning myocardium, and the quoted figure is approximately 40% of functioning myocardium, then the prognosis is grave. If the antegrade flow down the infarct-related vessel can be restored promptly, either by thrombolysis or direct angioplasty, then the incidence of shock may be reduced. Assuming that cardiogenic shock becomes established, treatment consists of the administration of inotropic drugs such as dobutamine and dopamine, diuretics and nitrates to reduce filling pressure, and often the use of intra-aortic balloon counter pulsation. Whereas these measures may produce a temporary improvement, they are not curative and it may prove impossible to wean the patient from the drugs or the balloon pump without repeated deterioration. Emergency cardiac transplantation has occasionally been used in this situation, but, of course, the scarcity of donors make this impractical to be used on a wide scale. Nevertheless, many interventional cardiologists would regard an acute anterior infarction complicated by cardiogenic shock as an indication for primary angioplasty.

Mitral regurgitation

Infarction or ischemia of the papillary muscle of the mitral valve apparatus can lead to mitral regurgitation. There is a wide spectrum in this condition. One extreme is frank papillary muscle rupture which leads to immediate hemodynamic compromise, acute pulmonary edema and often sudden death. Acute mitral regurgitation is poorly tolerated, unlike the situation in chronic rheumatic mitral regurgitation, where the left atrium has time to dilate and to become compliant and absorb a large regurgitant volume without a rise in pulmonary capillary wedge pressure. In acute mitral regurgitation, the wedge pressure rises dramatically and can cause acute pulmonary edema. At the other end of the spectrum is a subtle disruption of the complex mitral valve architecture comprising the valve and subvalve apparatus. This may produce a murmur of mitral regurgitation with only fairly mild hemodynamic disturbance or no hemodynamic disturbance at all. The frequency of mitral regurgitation varies according to how it is diagnosed, according to the published series. The reported incidence is between 10% and 55%. In a large series of 11 000 angiograms with documented postinfarction mitral regurgitation, the condition was an independent predictor of survival only when the regurgitation was moderate or severe, which occurred in only 3%. Overwhelming mitral regurgitation only occurs in about one out of six patients with the condition. Intra-aortic balloon pumping and the combination of inotropic agents and vasodilators may lead to hemodynamic improvement and enable the patient to be made fit for operation. Results would suggest that surgical intervention is better than medical therapy for severe mitral regurgitation, although the fact that many of these patients have severely impaired left ventricular function in addition to mitral regurgitation means that the surgical mortality is higher than for other causes of mitral regurgitation and is up to 41% in some series.

Myocardial rupture

Myocardial rupture can occur in up to 10% of fatal transmural infarctions and is a cause of sudden unheralded death. Attempts at resuscitation may be unsuccessful and electromechanical dissociation is one feature associated with this condition. Rupture of the free wall is associated with massive hemopericardium and tamponade. It appears to be more common in women than in men, and more common in hypertensives and in patients over the age of 60. In a large postmortem series described by Reddy and Roberts, 204 out of 648 postmortem hearts (31%) demonstrated a myocardial rupture and 67% of these involved the free wall and only 27% the intraventricular septum. Rupture of both occurred in 4%. Pathologically, it appears to be a stuttering, progressive process characterized by an infiltrating mural hemorrhage in a tear more than 1 day old. In patients who survive a myocardial rupture, a left ventricular false aneurysm may be produced. Here a rupture is contained by pericardial adhesions and a false aneurysm with a narrow neck is produced. The wall of the aneurysm is made up of pericardial elements and, within the aneurysm, clots may form and the aneurysm itself may rupture. The demonstration of a false left ventricular aneurysm is an indication for urgent resection because of the high risk of rupture. Echocardiography and radionuclide ventriculography, as well as more recently magnetic resonance imaging, have been shown to be able to detect these false aneurysms with a high degree of accuracy. It has been suggested that thrombolytic therapy makes myocardial rupture more likely but there is no sound evidence that this is true.

Rupture of the interventricular septum

Rupture of the interventricular septum as a consequence of myocardial infarction may produce a significant left-to-right shunt with the syndrome of cardiogenic shock and pulmonary edema. The murmur produced by rupture of the interventricular septum may be similar to that produced by acute mitral regurgitation, although its radiation tends to be towards the right-hand side of the sternum rather than to the axilla. The insertion of a Swan–Ganz balloon-tipped catheter into the right heart should enable one to differentiate between the two conditions. In mitral regurgitation, there may well be a large systolic V-wave on the pulmonary capillary wedge trace and the oxygen saturations in the right atrium, right ventricle and pulmonary artery will be the same. In ventricular septal rupture there will be a 'step-up' in saturations between the right atrium and the pulmonary artery as oxygenated blood enters the right ventricle and mixes with venous blood. Patients with acute ventricular septal rupture are often in extremis and intra-aortic balloon pumping coupled with inotropic agents and vasodilators will often produce hemodynamic improvement. The incidence of ventricular septal rupture appears to be much smaller than rupture of the free wall, as mentioned above, and a series of studies published between 1938 and 1968 show that only 7% of myocardial ruptures involved the septum, whereas 93% involved the free wall. The study of Reddy and Roberts suggested a somewhat higher incidence of ventricular septal rupture, as mentioned above. Until fairly recently, the management was to try and control the patient with balloon pumping, inotropic drugs and vasodilators for several weeks to enable the margins of the rupture to become more fibrous and give the surgical sutures a better chance of holding. The current practice is to opt for early surgery and there are many reports of excellent results from early repair of ventricular septal defects. Again, echocardiography and color flow Doppler may demonstrate the site of the ventricular septal rupture very well, and in some patients cardiac catheterization is not necessary to delineate the site of the rupture or to calculate the size of the shunt. The only purpose of doing a coronary angiogram is to define the coronary anatomy so that coronary bypass grafting can be carried out at the same time.

True ventricular aneurysms

The definition of a ventricular aneurysm has been the subject of some debate. Angiographically, it is characterized by a large anteroapical akinetic segment which may or may not exhibit paradoxical motion during systole. However, not all such appearances on angiograms will be found to be aneurysmal at the time of surgery, and some of these so-called aneurysms may in fact contain viable myocardium. A true ventricular aneurysm consists of a thinned expanded area of myocardium which has been replaced by fibrous tissue. They may often be responsible for left ventricular failure, and be associated with cardiac arrhythmias and mural thrombus (see below). If the non-aneurysmal segment of ventricle is very vigorous the patient may be totally asymptomatic and the presence of an aneurysm *per se* is not an indication for surgical intervention. True ventricular aneurysms with a wall of fibrous tissue do not rupture. If a non-aneurysmal segment is not vigorous, the patient may be short of breath on exertion or have attacks of pulmonary edema, but even under these circumstances the results of left ventricular aneurysmectomy are not wonderful.

Pericarditis

Pericardial rub is common after a myocardial infarction and pericardial pain can be differentiated from ischemic pain by its relationship to inspiration or posture, although the character of the pain may be very similar to pain of the infarction. ST segment elevation of a pericarditic nature may occur in the infarct-related leads or in remote leads. More often than not, a pericarditis requires no more than treatment with analgesics and anti-inflammatories and is usually self-limiting. More rarely, a condition known as Dressler's syndrome may occur which is characterized by a fever, a pericardial and/or pleural rub and effusions, and anemia. The incidence of this in some series is as high as 4% and is usually a single self-limiting episode which responds to anti-inflammatories or possibly steroids. Rarely, constrictive pericarditis can occur following an effusion related to Dressler's syndrome. Antimyocardial antibodies can be demonstrated in some cases, but whether these are causal is be no means proven.

Mural thrombus

Mural thrombus nearly always complicates anterior rather than inferior myocardial infarction and the clot is usually situated at the apex of the left ventricle. It can be demonstrated on echocardiography, magnetic resonance imaging or by contrast angiography, although the latter is probably less sensitive than the echocardiogram. Mural thrombus is a source of potential emboli including strokes and 1.5–3.6% of patients with anterior infarction suffer strokes which are thought to be embolic in nature. There is a strong correlation between the demonstration of mural thrombus and the risk of embolization, and anticoagulation with warfarin reduces the risk of stroke. Some cardiologists routinely anticoagulate patients with impaired left ventricular function, even if thrombus cannot be demonstrated by any imaging technique.

Ongoing ischemia postinfarction

It is quite common for patients to experience ischemic pain on and off for the first 24 hours after a myocardial infarction, and this nearly always settles with the use of intravenous nitrates and heparin. The patient may or may not experience ECG changes associated with the pain. Threatened reocclusion after thrombolysis with ST segment elevation in the infarct-related leads may require a second dose of thrombolytic therapy and, if the patient has received streptokinase initially, then tissue plasminogen activator may be given the second time. Ongoing ischemia, despite these measures, will provoke early investigation with a view to angioplasty or bypass surgery.

Myocardial stunning and hibernation

Stunning and hibernation are two relatively new concepts in cardiology. Myocardial stunning is characterized by post ischemic left ventricular dysfunction which is likely to recover spontaneously. In other words, the demonstration of akinesis or hypokinesis after a severe ischemic insult does not necessarily imply that such hypokinesis is irreversible. Metabolic alterations in stunned myocardium have been demonstrated using positron emission tomography and [^{11}C]acetate and [^{11}C]palmitate studies have shown that stunned myocardium demonstrates reduced fatty acid and overall oxidative metabolism which gradually normalizes over time. As myocardial metabolism normalizes, so does regional function. Recovery to normal contractility may be delayed for hours, days or even weeks. It is thus dangerous to use the assessment of left ventricular function too early after ischemic insult in order to decide whether a segment is worthy of revascularization or not. Some studies have suggested that calcium antagonists may be beneficial and protect against postischemic stunning.

Hibernating myocardium is hypothesized to be a state where the myocytes are 'down-regulated' in response to prolonged hypoperfusion that may last for weeks or months, yet this myocardium retains the potential for functional recovery after revascularization. In myocardial hibernation, blood flow and cardiac function are once again in equilibrium, so that neither myocardial necrosis nor ischemic symptoms may be present. Hibernating myocardium has been demonstrated to occur with unstable angina, chronic stable angina, myocardial infarction and, most importantly, with left ventricular dysfunction and congestive cardiac failure. Before the concept of myocardial hibernation became accepted, several studies were published on the effects of coronary bypass surgery on so-called 'bad ventricles'. The different results in these studies may have been partly related to the fact that ventricles that improved after revascularization in fact contained hibernating myocardium, whereas those that did not contained infarcted irreversibly damaged myocardium. It is important clinically to recognize hibernating myocardium. Studies have shown that patients with hibernating myocardium who are revascularized have a much lower incidence of cardiac death than those who are not revascularized, indicating that the salvage of hibernating myocardium is important in improving survival.

Myocardial viability

It is not possible to detect by angiographic appearances whether akinetic or hypokinetic appearances are due to scar or hibernation. Positron emission tomography can demonstrate continued metabolic activity in areas that are chronically underperfused. Areas of myocardium that demonstrate reduced flow, either by thallium scintigraphy or by using [^{13}N]ammonia, but demonstrate continued metabolic activity either with [^{18}F]fluorine deoxyglucose or with [^{11}C]palmitate, are areas that are hibernating. Areas of myocardium that demonstrate both absent or diminished flow and absent metabolism are not likely to benefit from revascularization. Unfortunately, positron emission tomography is not widely available, but uptake of thallium-201 at rest is a moderately good indicator of myocardial viability. When assessing patients for myocardial viability, it is important to assess myocardial blood flow under true resting conditions. It is, therefore, not sufficient to carry out an exercise thallium scan followed by delayed imaging 4 hours later, which indicates what has happened during the redistribution period. The reason for this is that, if an area is profoundly ischemic, the thallium may not have redistributed into the myocardium within 4 hours and give the interpreter of the image a false impression. The current trend is, therefore, to carry out a stress image followed either by reinjection on the same day or reinjection at a later date. By reinjecting thallium, say 24 hours later, one can assess what the myocardium is like under true resting conditions.

Unusual causes of myocardial infarction

Finally, it is worth mentioning some of the more unusual causes of myocardial infarction. Dissection of a coronary artery can occur as a consequence of aortic root dissection, for example, in patients with Marfan's syndrome or in hypertensives, and spontaneous coronary artery dissection has also been reported, particularly during pregnancy. Coronary arteries can also be dissected at the time of catheterization or during angioplasty, which can lead to myocardial infarction.

Autoimmune diseases such as systemic lupus erythematosus can produce a coronary arteritis which can lead to coronary occlusion. Some patients with systemic lupus have circulating anticardiolipin antibody which may predispose to premature coronary thrombosis.

Myocardial contusion can also produce infarction. The example shown in Figure 202 is of a karate student who developed acute ischemic chest pain after closed chest trauma during practice. He had evidence of myocardial necrosis on scintigraphic grounds and on enzyme criteria.

Myocardial infarction can also occur the arteries of a transplanted heart, and coronary artery disease is the commonest cause of death 1 year after cardiac transplantation. Syphilitic aortitis is uncommon nowadays but can involve the coronary ostia and produce coronary occlusion. Pheochromocytoma can produce myocardial infarction during hypertensive crises. Finally, myocardial infarction is not unknown in patients who have angiographically normal coronary arteries, even in the absence of obvious coagulation problems such as protein C deficiency or the presence of the circulating lupus anticoagulant.

Section 2 Myocardial Infarction Illustrated

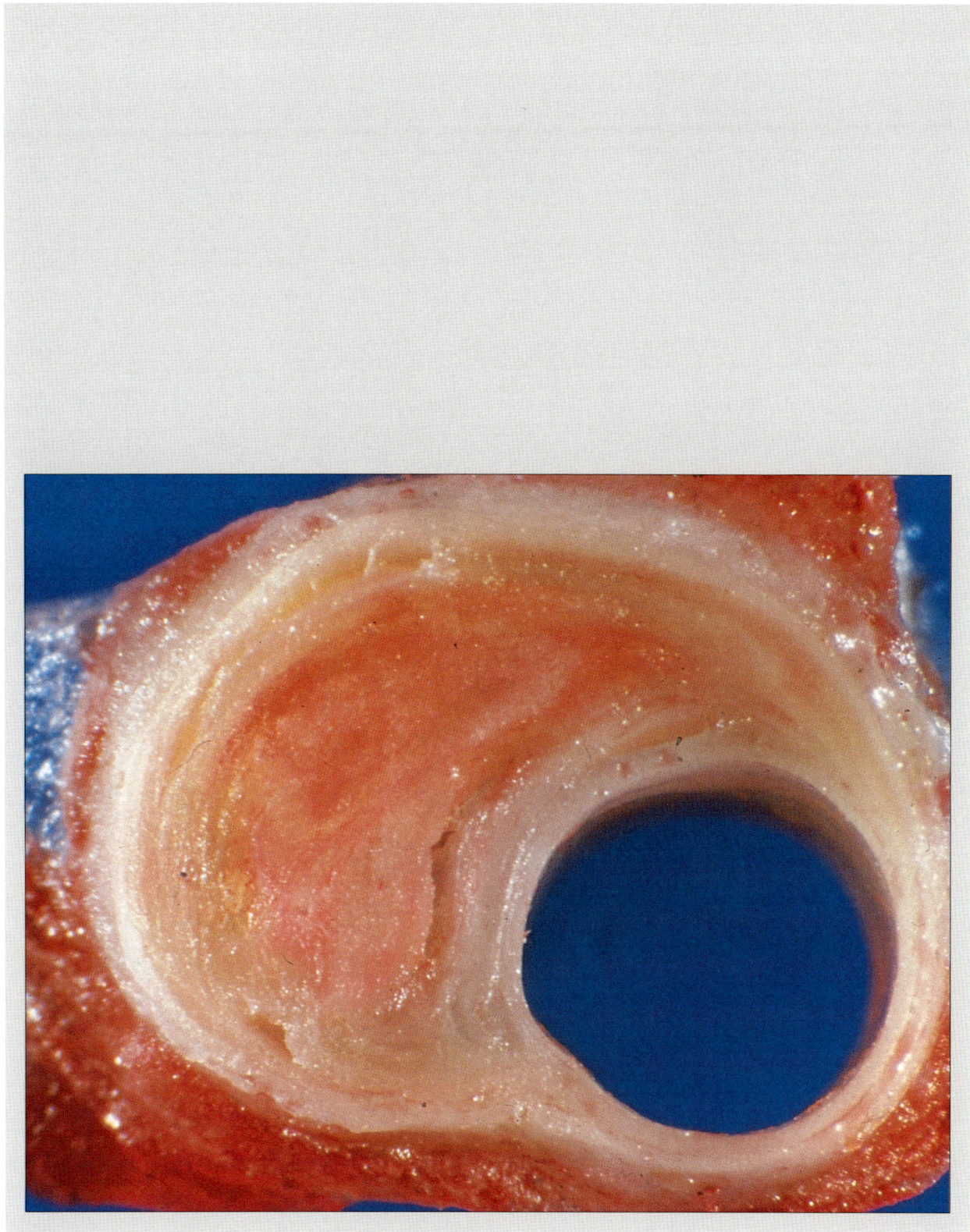

Figure 1 Cut end of human coronary artery stained for
lipid with oil-red O. Pericardial fat stains bright red and the
large plaque is rich in pink-stained lipid

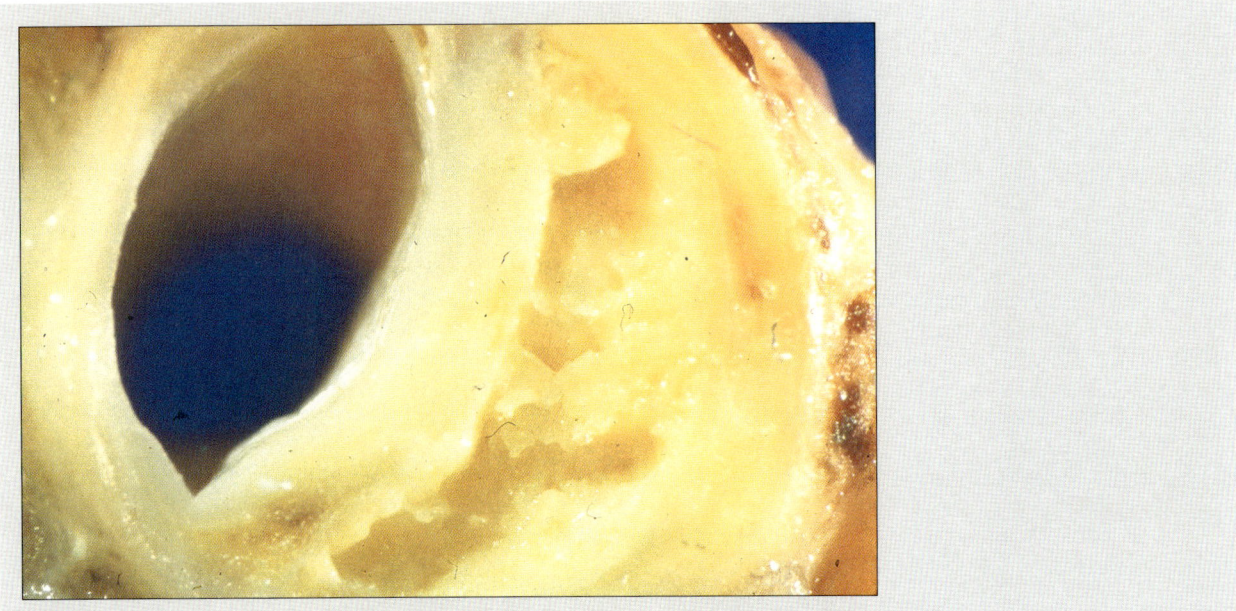

Figure 2 Unstained cut end of human coronary artery showing a very large lipid-rich plaque with a significant but not critical stenosis obstructing the lumen

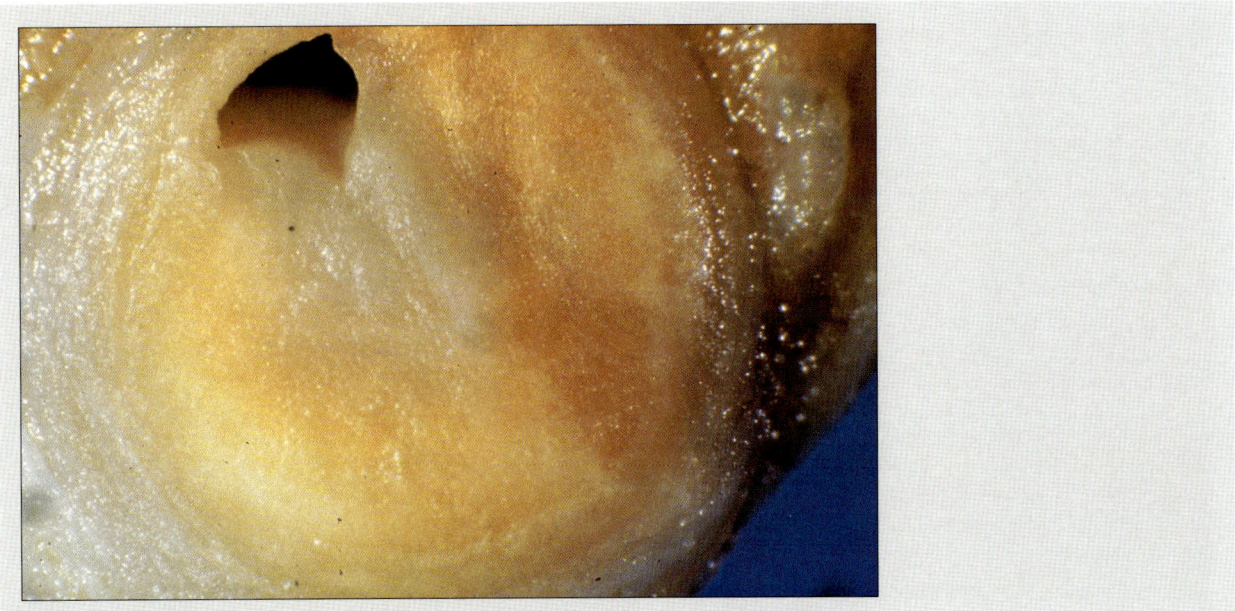

Figure 3 Cut end of human coronary artery showing a large lipid-rich plaque with an extremely tight stenosis restricting the lumen. The section is unstained. There is no thrombus. This is from a patient with familial hypercholesterolemia

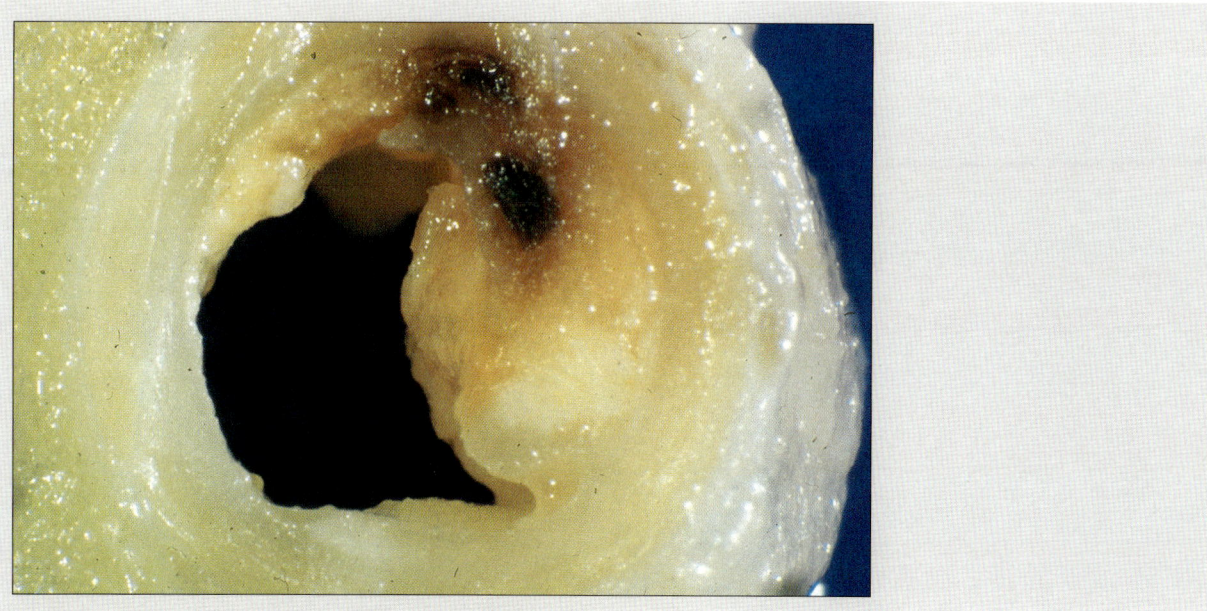

Figure 4 Cut end of human coronary artery showing a lipid-rich plaque with some disruption. The lipid-rich content is mixed with thrombus but there is no clot obstructing the lumen. This is taken from a patient who had presented previously with unstable angina

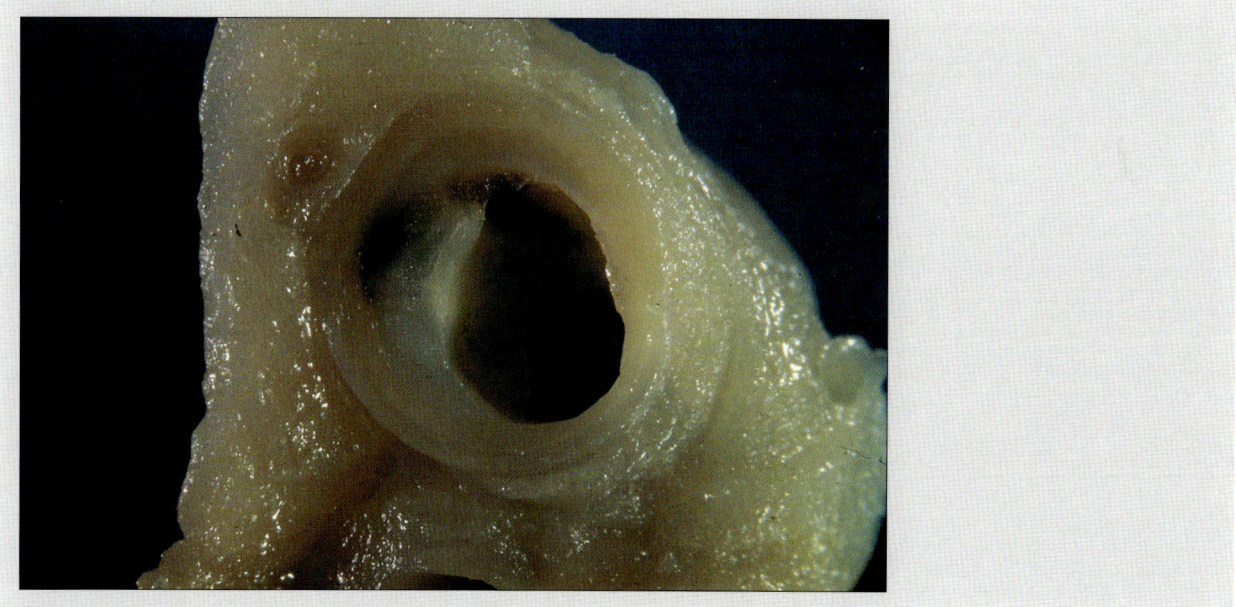

Figure 5 Cut end of human coronary artery showing a plaque which is unstained but with thrombus becoming organized into the plaque. There is also some fibrous tissue which appears less yellow

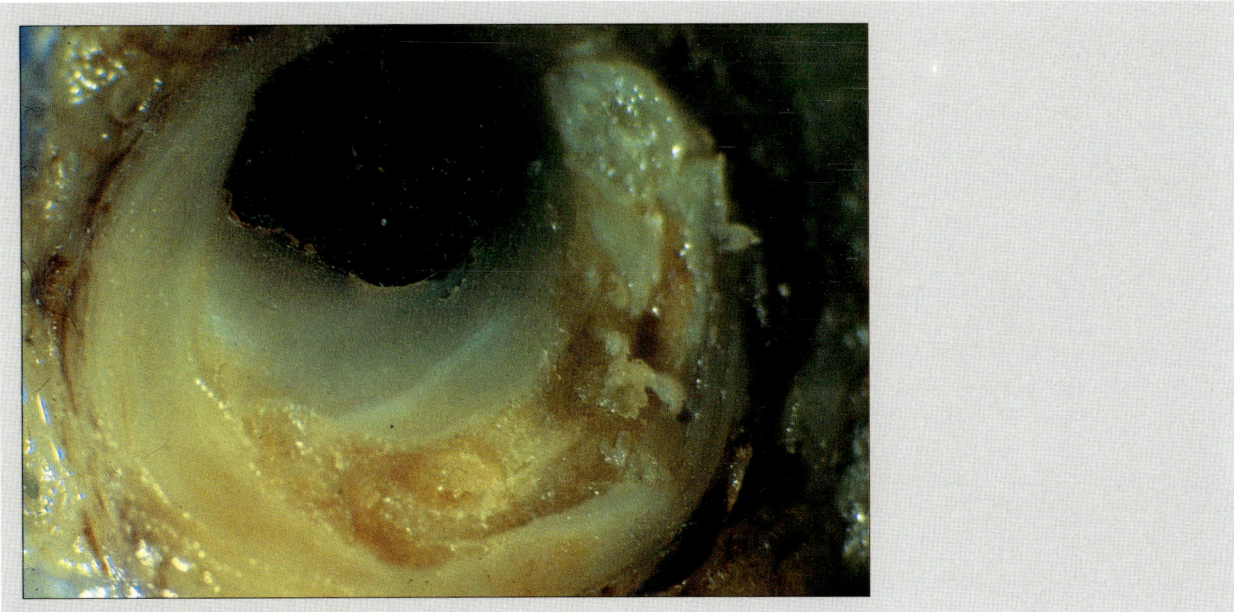

Figure 6 Cut end of human coronary artery showing a large lipid-rich plaque in yellow over which thrombus has occluded the vessel

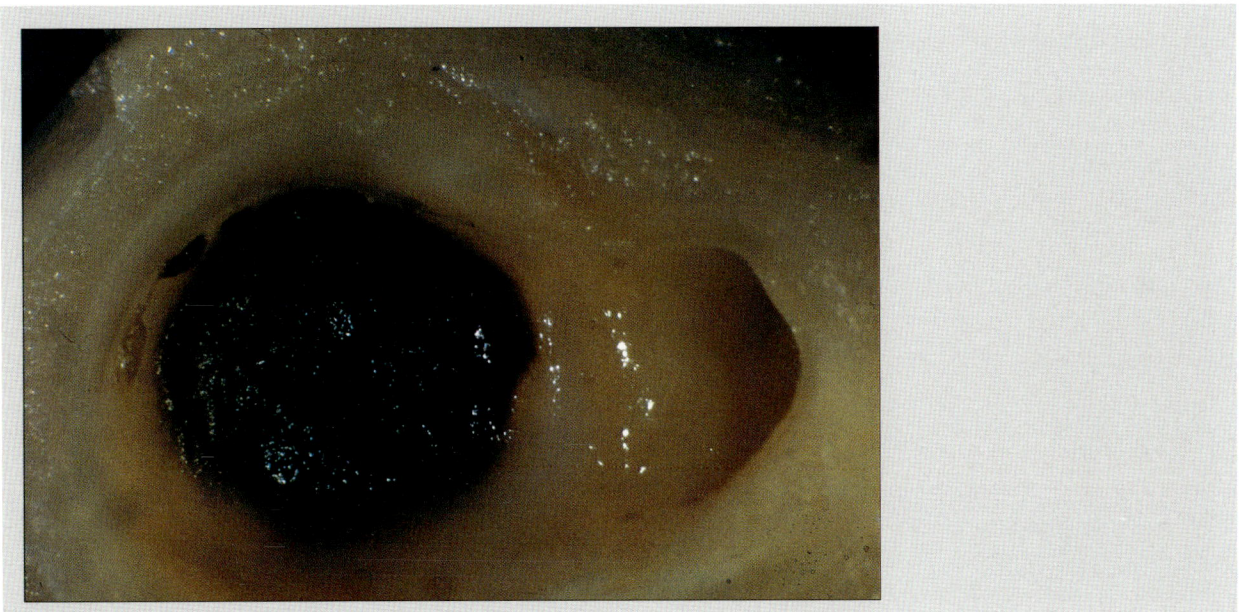

Figure 7 Cut end of human coronary artery showing massive occlusive thrombus just beyond the origin of a side branch which is seen to the right. The side branch is spared

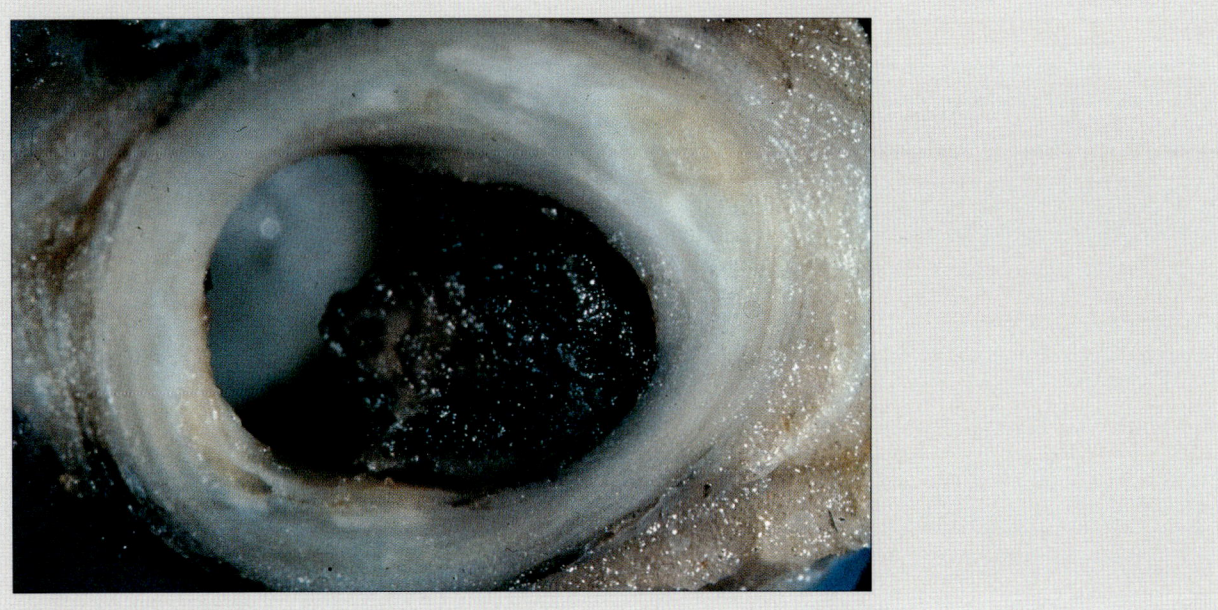

Figure 8 Cut end of human coronary artery showing a large but non-occlusive thrombus. This is the sort of situation one associates with a non-Q wave infarction or unstable or crescendo angina

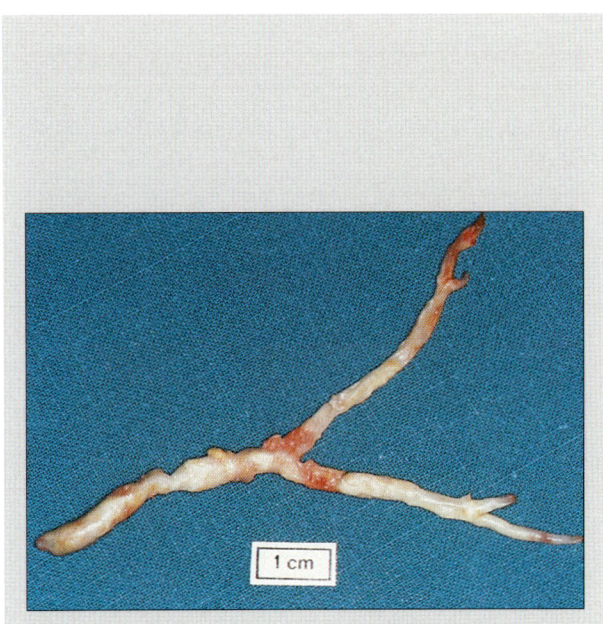

Figure 9 Operative specimen of right coronary artery atheroma removed surgically during an endarterectomy. The vessel was totally occluded with this atheroma

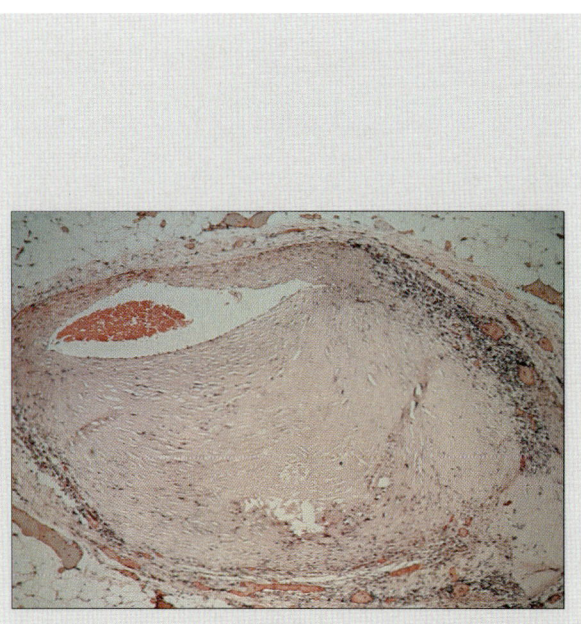

Figure 10 Histological section showing a cross-section of a large collagen plaque stained with hematoxylin and eosin. Note the adventitial inflammation in the top right-hand corner where there is intense macrophage infiltration

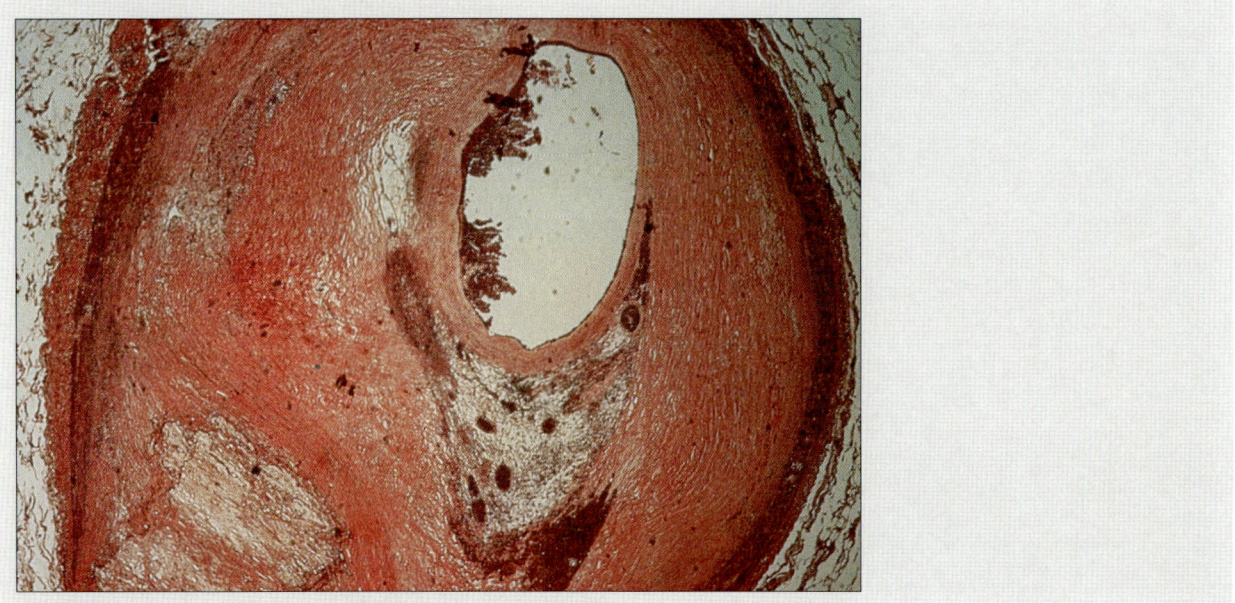

Figure 11 Histological cross-section of a large fibrous plaque using a van Giesen stain, which stains collagen red. Note the thrombus in more than one place inside the plaque which indicates that plaque rupture has occurred more than once

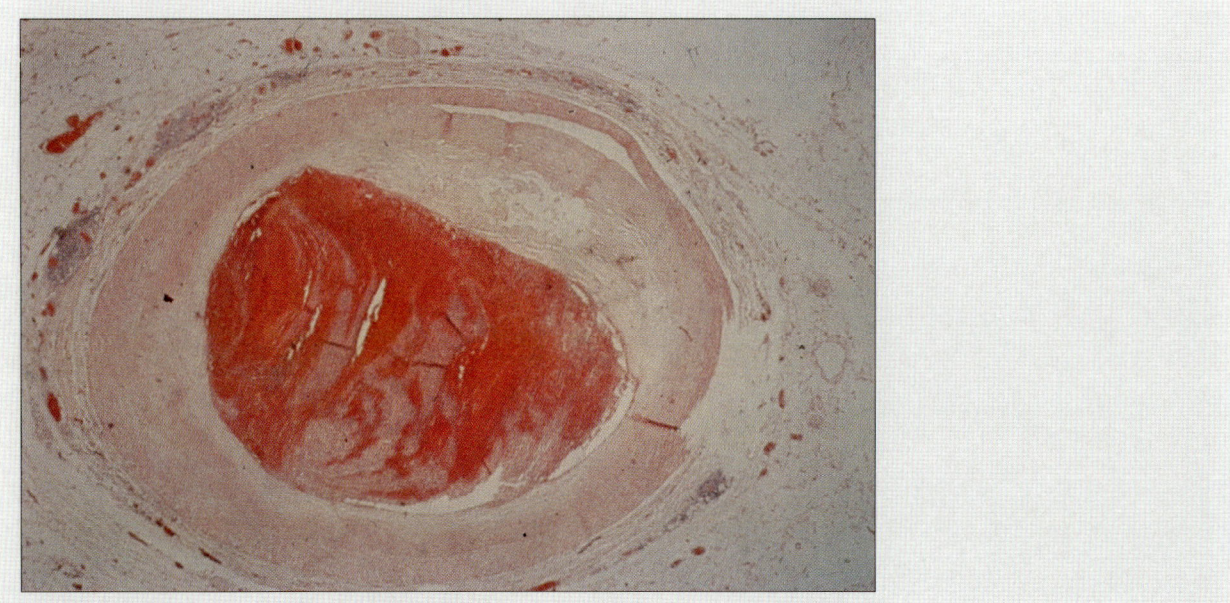

Figure 12 Histological cross-section of a human artery using a van Giesen stain. A large thrombus is seen obstructing the lumen

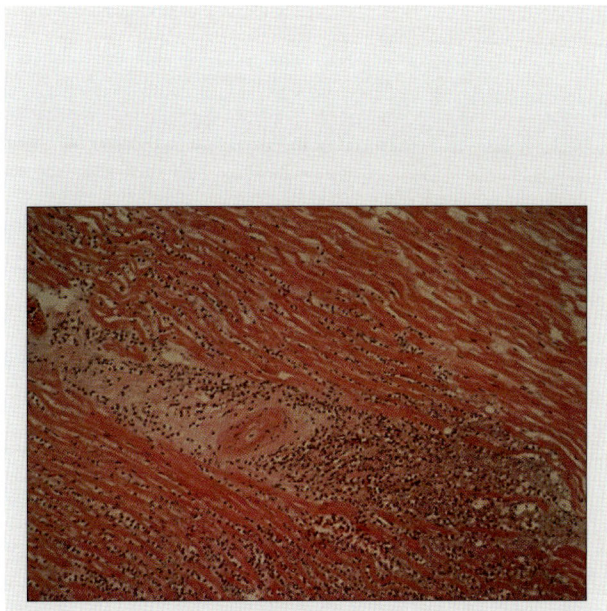

Figure 13 Microscopic section of heart muscle in the early stages of myocardial infarction. The section is stained with H & E stain. Note the intense polymorphonuclear leukocyte infiltration between the myocytes. This is the sort of appearance seen in the first 24 hours of infarction

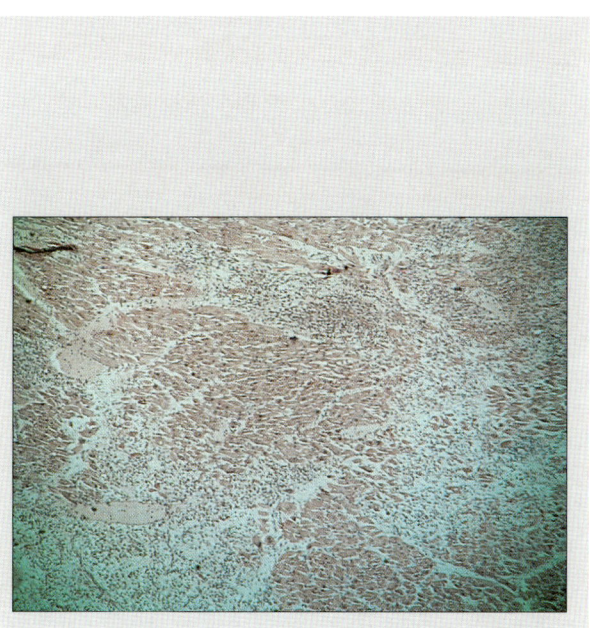

Figure 14 H & E stain of section of a 5-day old myocardial infarction. The surviving myocytes shown in reddish-brown are surrounded by macrophages and very few fibroblasts. This is the early stage of healing

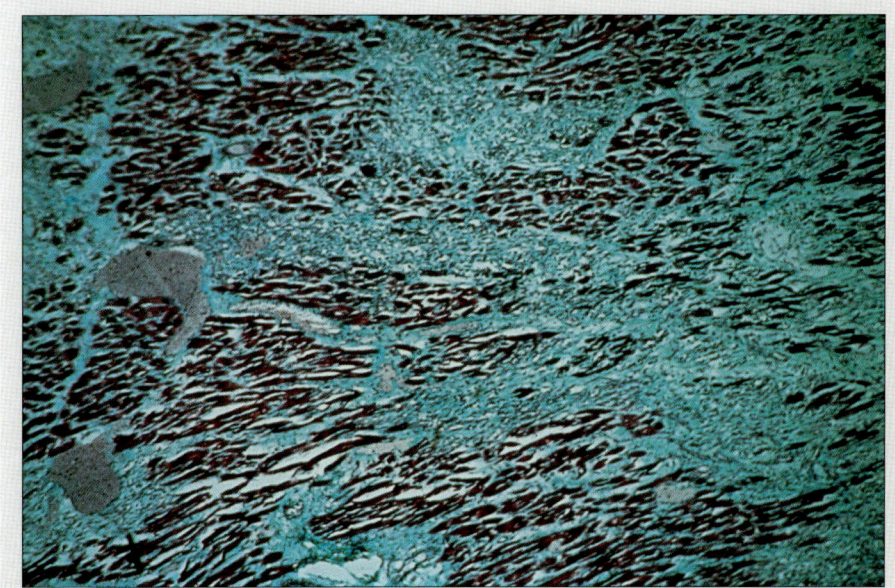

Figure 15 Trichrome stain where the surviving myocytes are shown in dark brown and swathes of collagen are shown in green. Note there are no macrophages. This infarction would be at least several weeks old

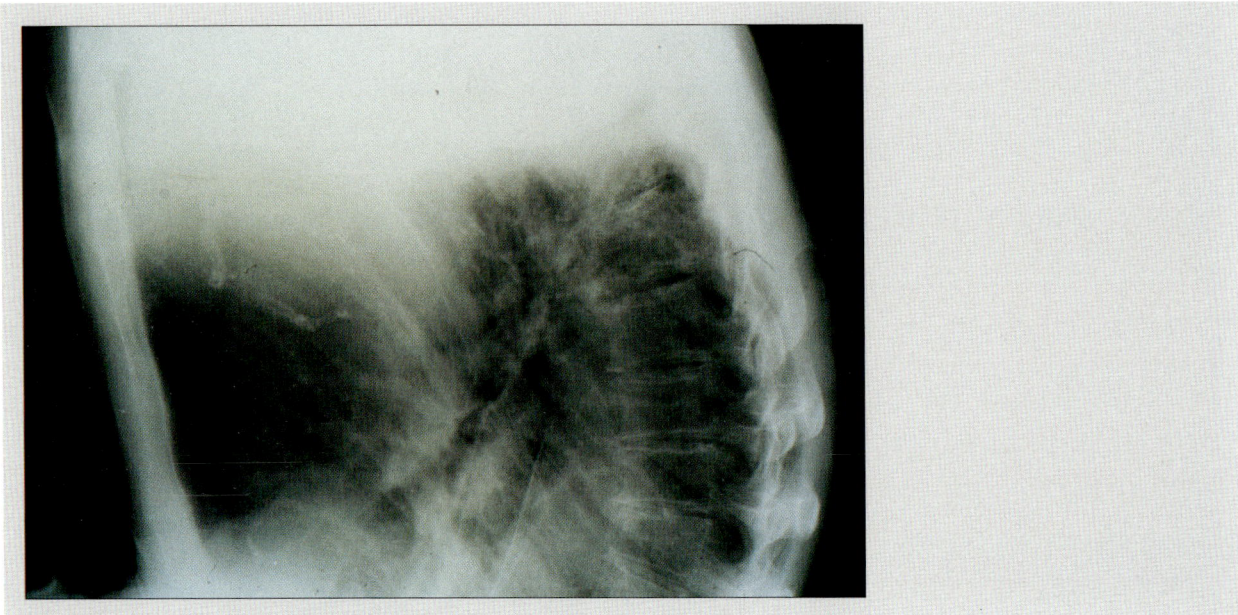

Figure 16 Left lateral chest X-ray showing calcification of the coronary arteries, which is a common finding in coronary atherosclerotic disease

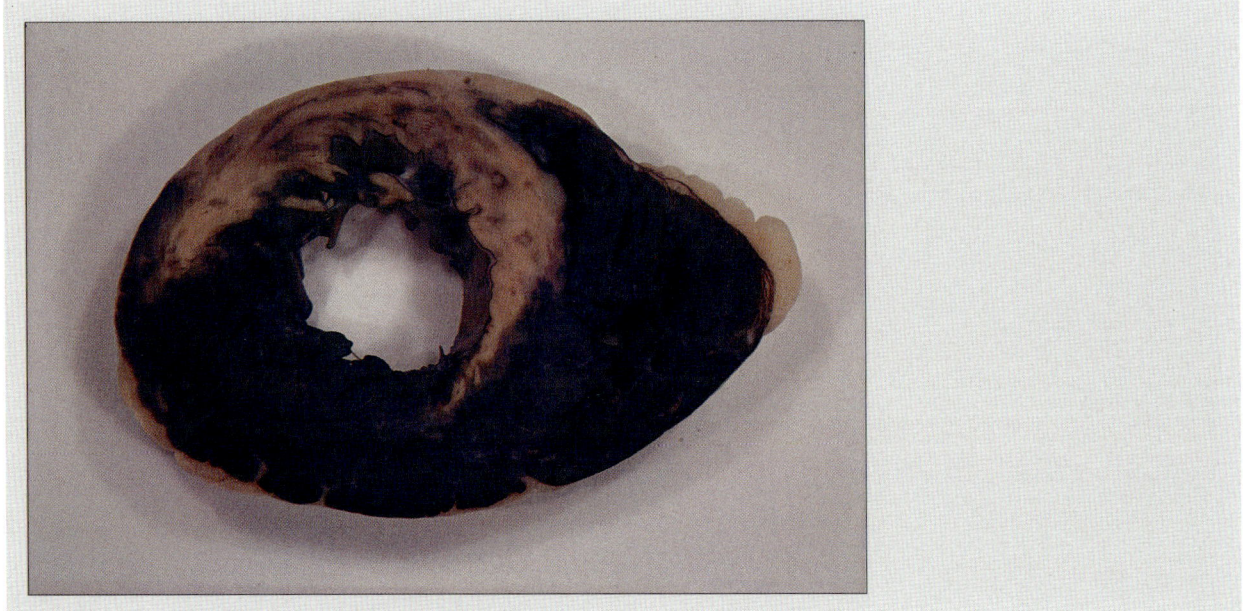

Figure 17 Postmortem heart cut in cross-section and stained for succinic dehydrogenase. Cells which are intact and contain the latter enzyme are shown as blue, whereas the areas that have lost the enzyme show up as white. Infarctions involving the anterior wall and the interventricular septum are shown as areas that have lost enzyme

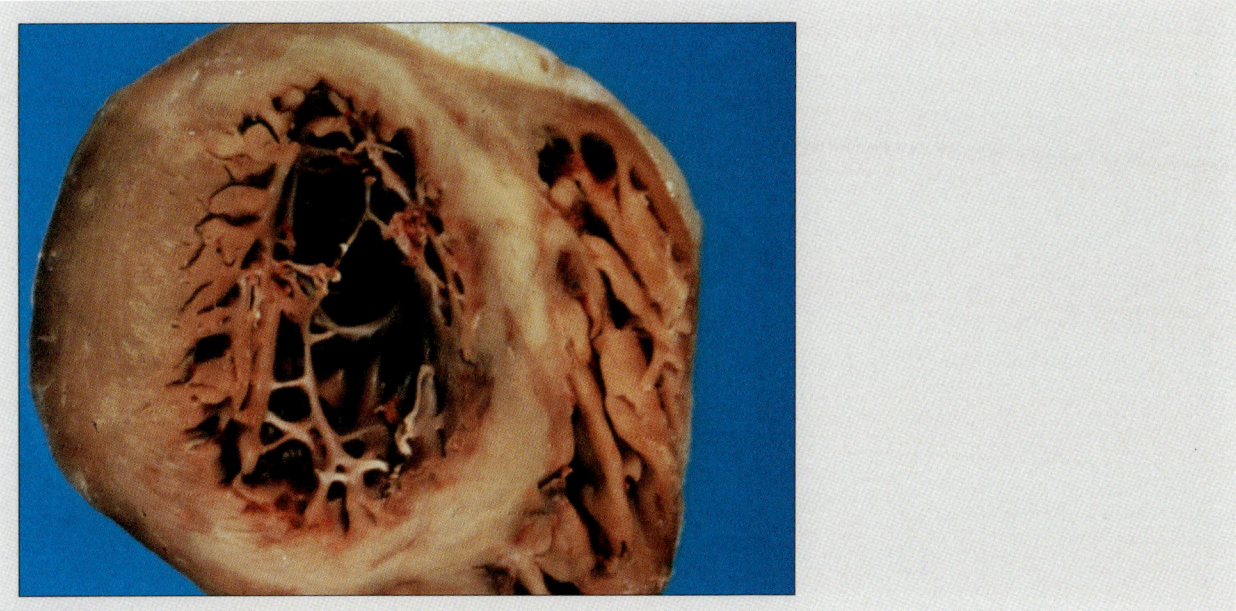

Figure 18 Cross-section of postmortem heart showing right and left ventricles. An old healed anteroseptal infarction is shown as the white area between the two ventricles

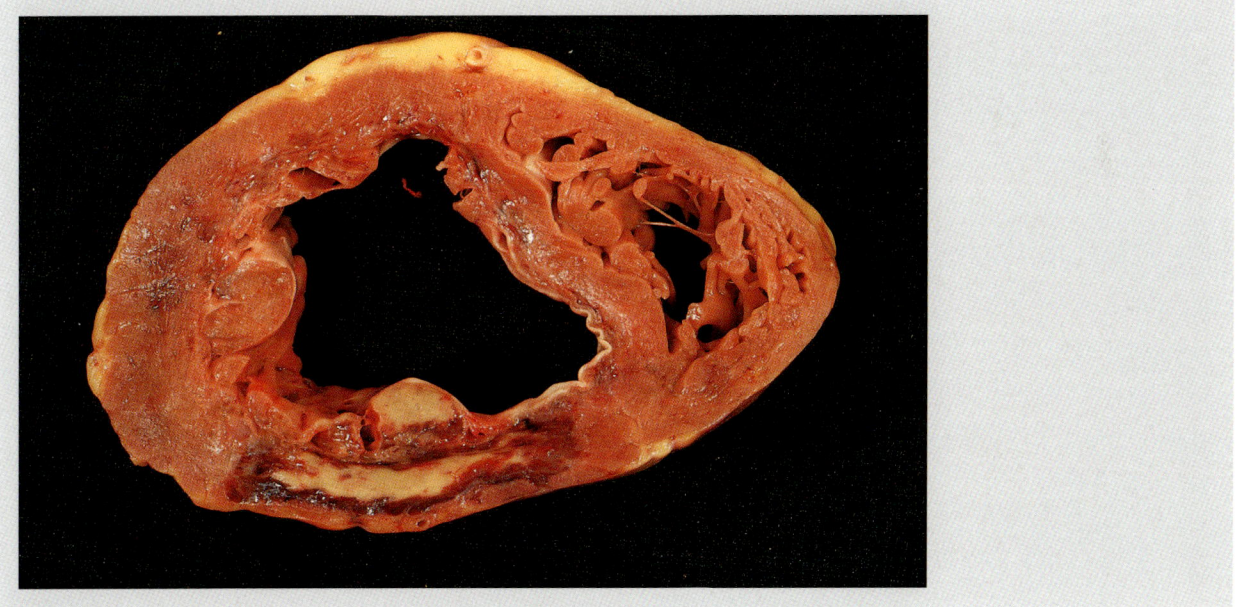

Figure 19 Short-axis cut of a postmortem heart showing a recent posterior infarction. The infarcted muscle is shown as bright yellow, with blood vessels and capillary-dense rim around the yellow area. Note the intact epicardium which is thought to protect the heart from infarct expansion

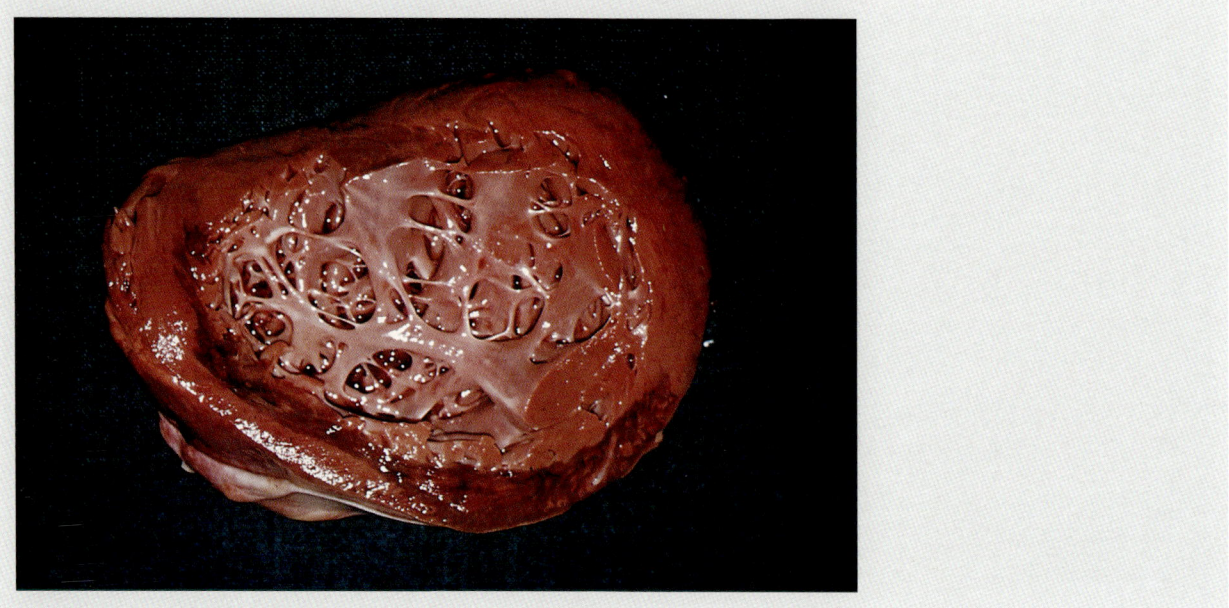

Figure 20 Postmortem heart showing a myocardial infarction as a red area with well-defined margins. The pericardium can be seen just below the infarct and peeled back

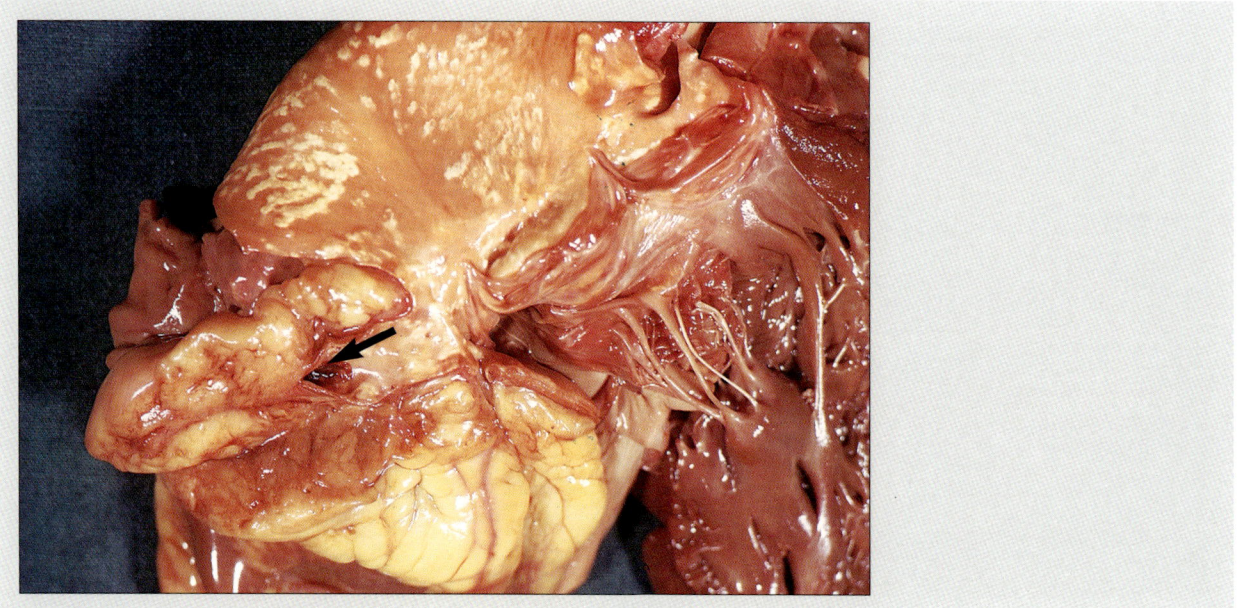

Figure 21 Postmortem heart showing the coronary artery opened on the left-hand side of the picture with fresh thrombus situated in the vessel (arrowed)

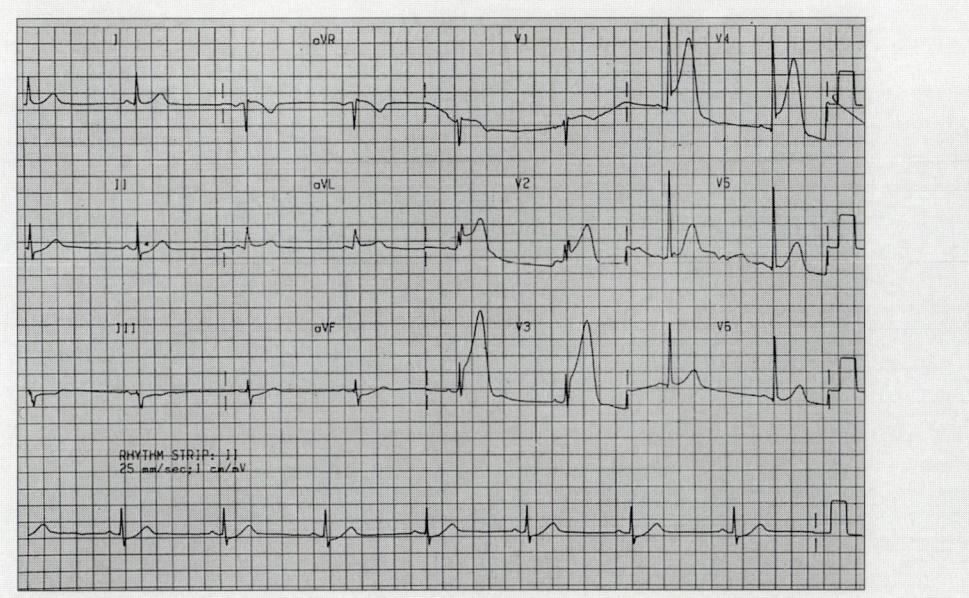

Figure 22 12-lead electrocardiogram from a patient 1½ hours into an acute anteroseptal myocardial infarction due to thrombotic occlusion of the left anterior descending coronary artery. Note the tall ST segment elevation in leads V2, V3 and V4

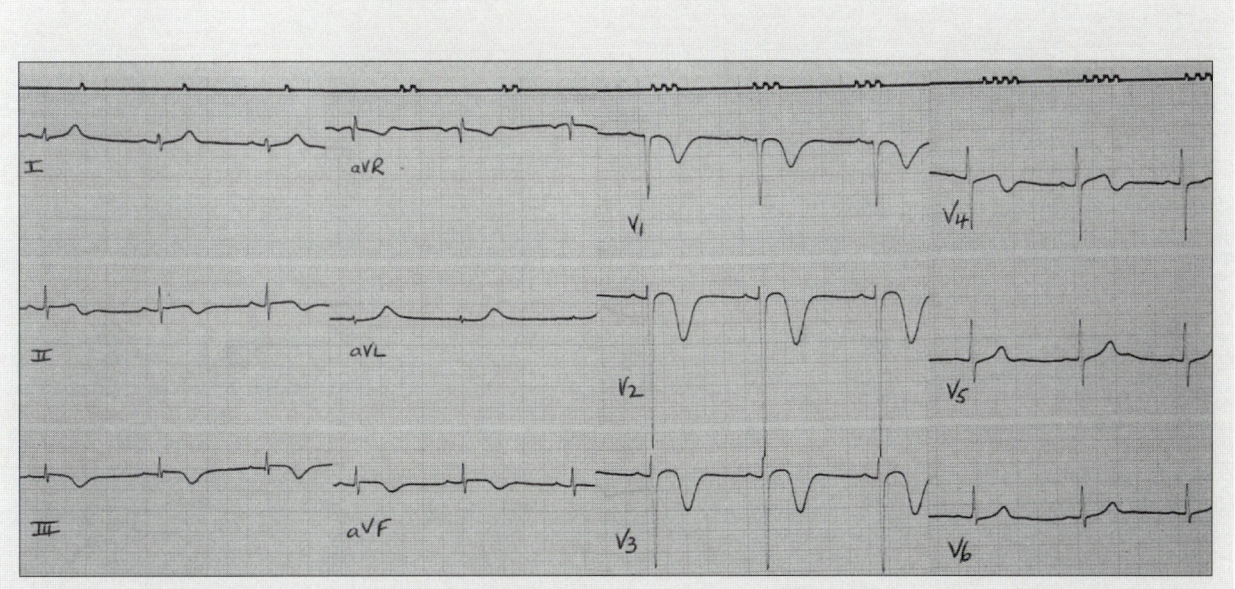

Figure 23 Same patient as in Figure 22 6 hours after the administration of thrombolytic therapy with intravenous tissue plasminogen activator. Note the deep symmetrical T wave inversion in leads V1–V4 with preservation of R-wave. There is also some inferior T wave inversion. These are the typical appearances of a non-Q wave myocardial infarction and indicate successful myocardial salvage

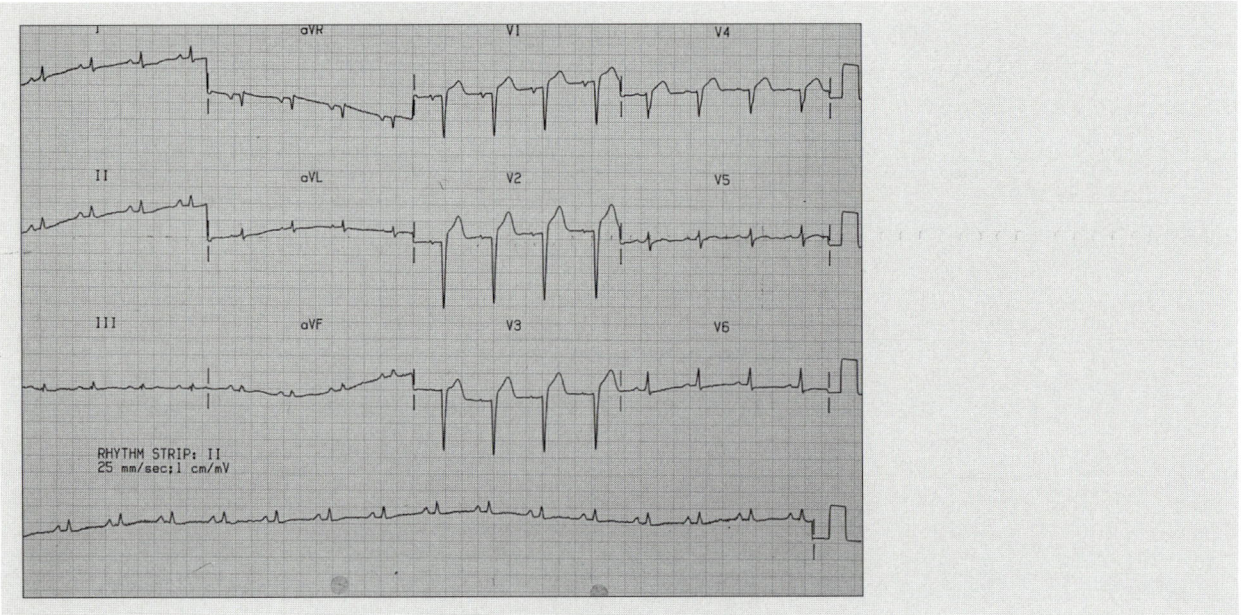

Figure 24 12-lead electrocardiogram from a patient who received streptokinase 6 hours into an acute anterior myocardial infarction. Although the pain promptly resolved, there are deep Q waves in leads V1–V4 with persistent ST segment elevation. This sometimes, but not always, indicates failed thrombolysis

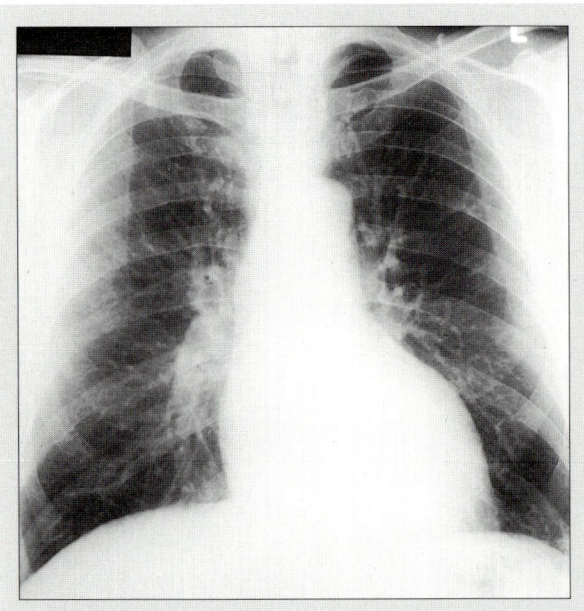

Figure 25 Posteroanterior chest X-ray from the same patient as in Figure 24 on the day of admission showing marked upper lobe pulmonary venous distension, indicating a raised pulmonary capillary wedge pressure and some degree of pulmonary edema. This is a more reliable sign for an indication to give diuretics than basal crepitations on auscultation

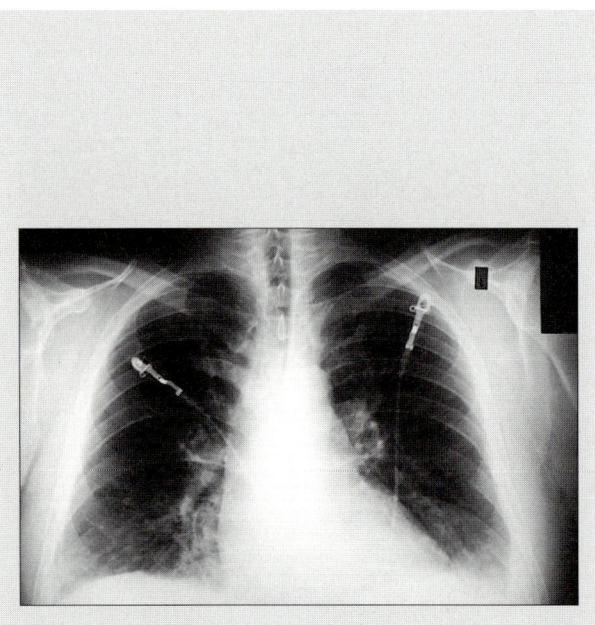

Figure 26 Posteroanterior chest X-ray from same patient as in Figures 24 and 25 48 hours after admission. The upper lobe veins are no longer distended after diuretic therapy

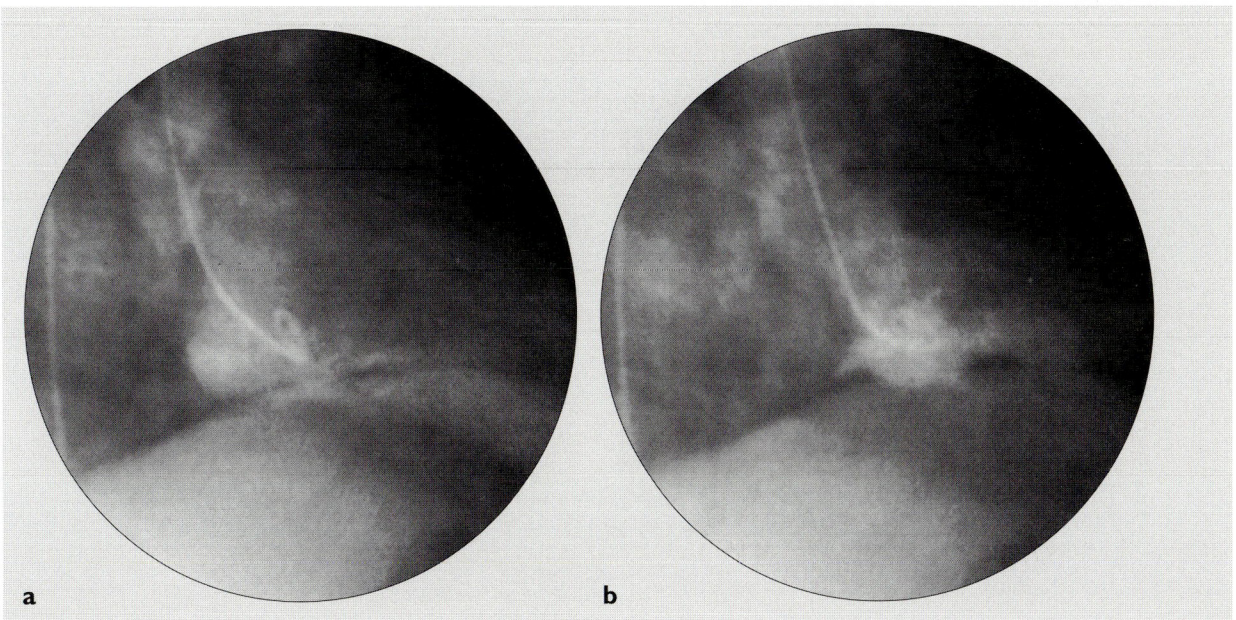

a   b

Figure 27 (a) End-diastolic frame and (b) end-systolic frame from the patient whose ECG is shown in Figure 24. Angiography was carried out 6 weeks after the initial event and, in spite of persistent Q waves, there is good overall left ventricular function and the anterior wall still moves

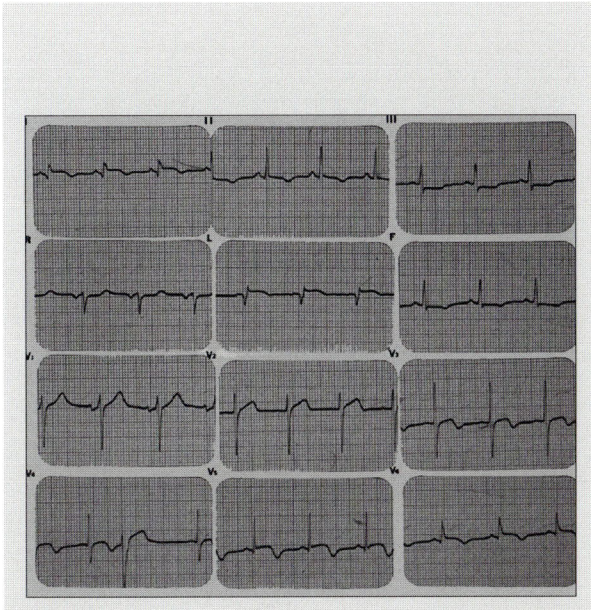

Figure 28 12-lead ECG of an anterolateral myocardial infarction with Q waves in leads I, AVL and V6, and T wave inversion in V3, V4 and V5. There are also some inferior ST segment changes

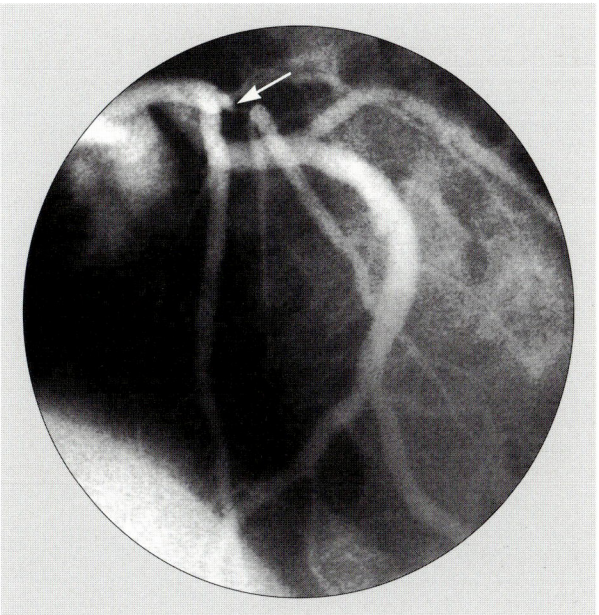

Figure 29 Coronary arteriogram from the same patient as in Figure 28 showing a subtotal occlusion of a large diagonal branch (arrowed). The left anterior descending branch is seen running vertically down the interventricular septum just beyond where the diagonal is subtotally occluded. The other large vessel is the circumflex which is dominant

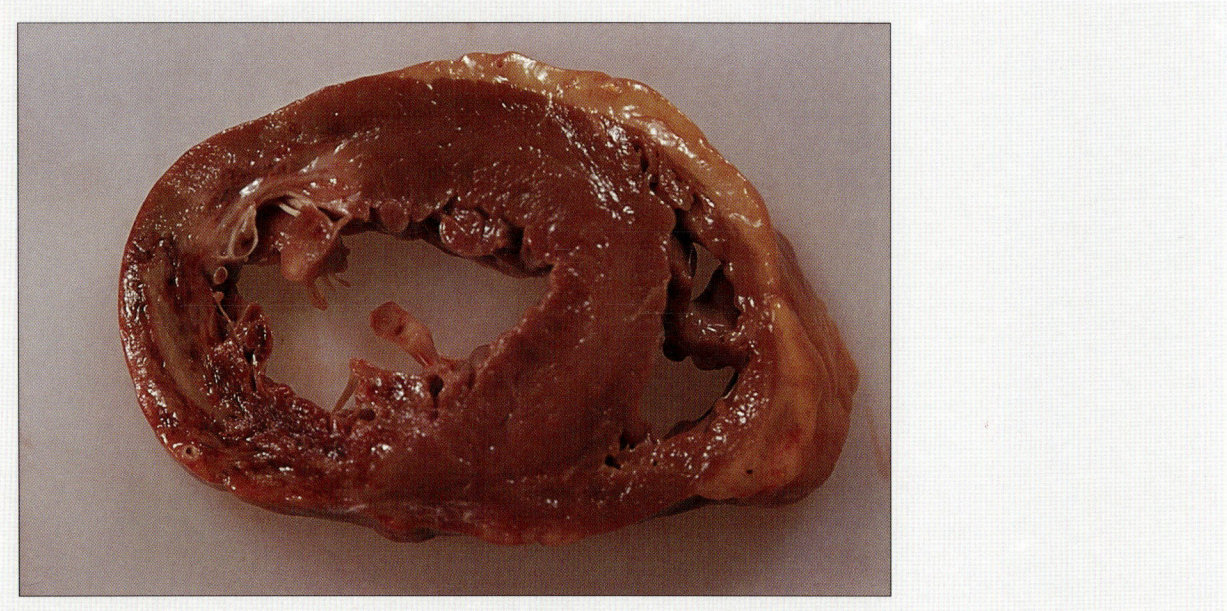

Figure 30 Postmortem specimen from a patient with a fresh lateral wall infarct. Note that the ventricular septum is intact between the right and left ventricles and the pale area on the free wall is the site of the lateral infarct

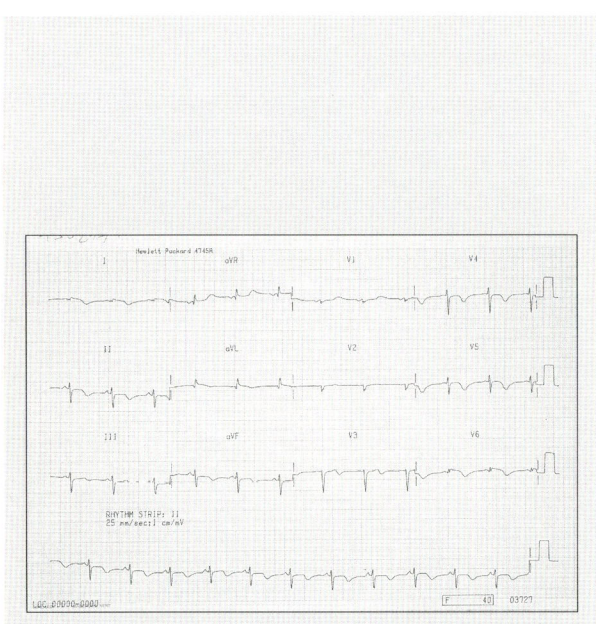

Figure 31 12-lead ECG from a patient with a non-Q wave inferolateral infarction due to a subtotal occlusion of a large circumflex vessel

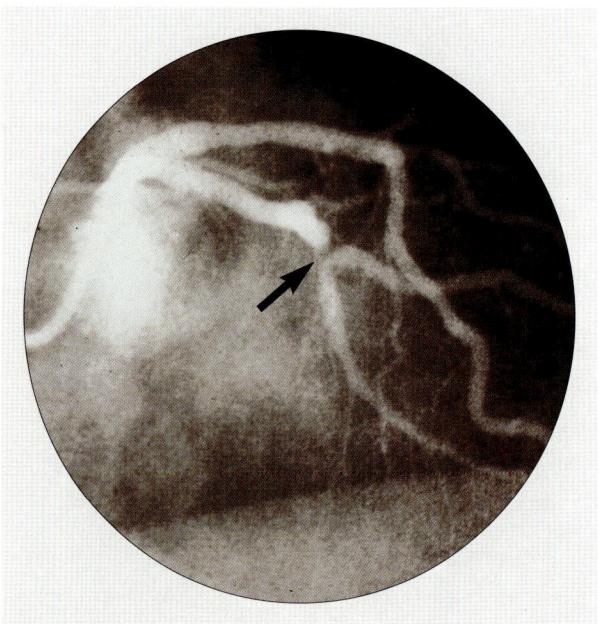

Figure 32 Coronary angiogram from same patient as in Figure 31 showing tight circumflex stenosis (arrowed)

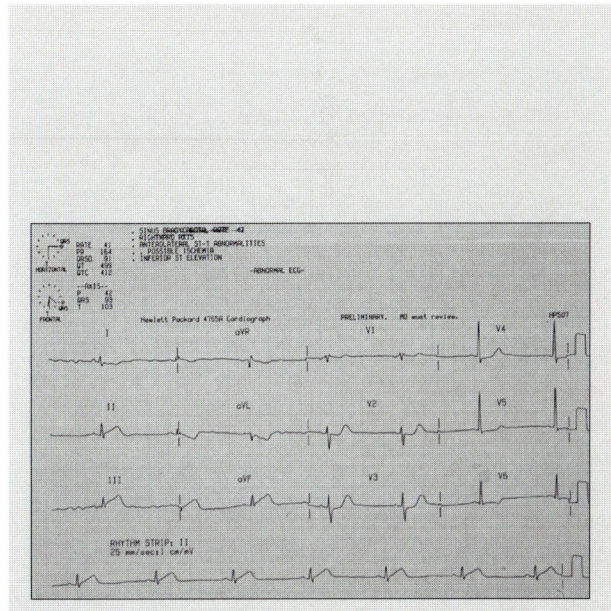

Figure 33 12-lead ECG from a patient 45 min into severe chest pain showing 'hyperacute' ST segment elevation in leads II, III and AVF. These changes, where the T wave seems to arise directly from the QRS segment, are typical of the very early infarction changes

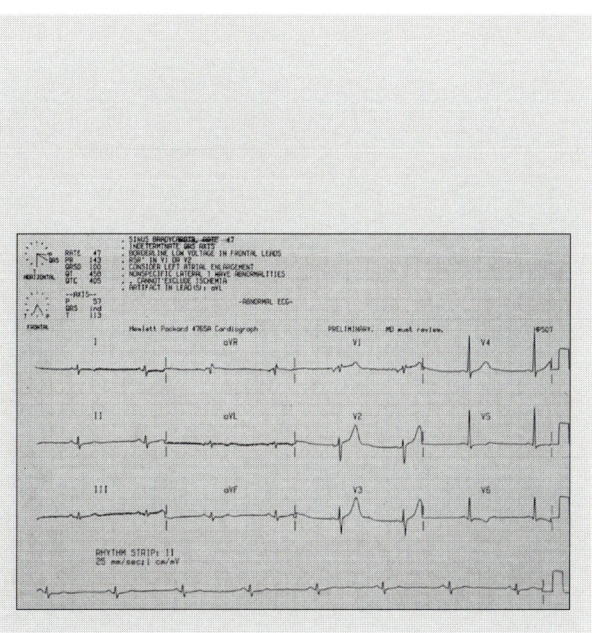

Figure 34 Same patient as in Figure 33 2 hours after streptokinase administration intravenously. The inferior changes have reverted to normal and there are some T wave changes in the lateral leads only

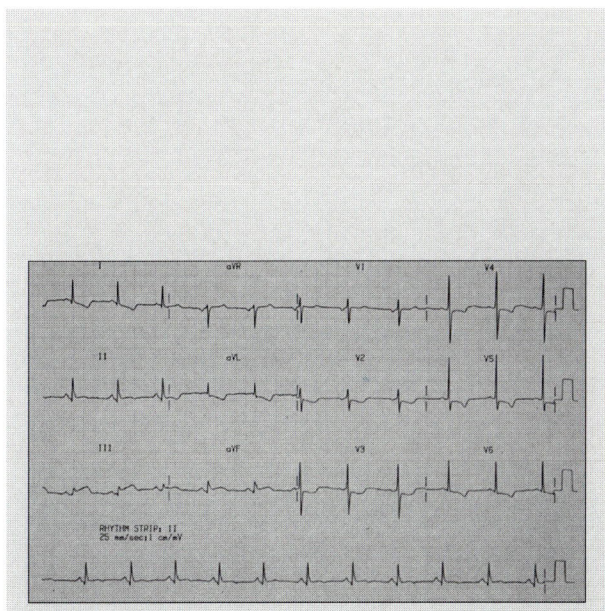

Figure 35 Acute ST segment elevation in leads II, III and AVF in a patient with a previous anterior myocardial infarction. Note the ST segment depression in leads V2 and V3 and T wave inversion in leads V4–V6. On the basis of one ECG alone, it is not possible to say whether these changes are 'reciprocal' or not

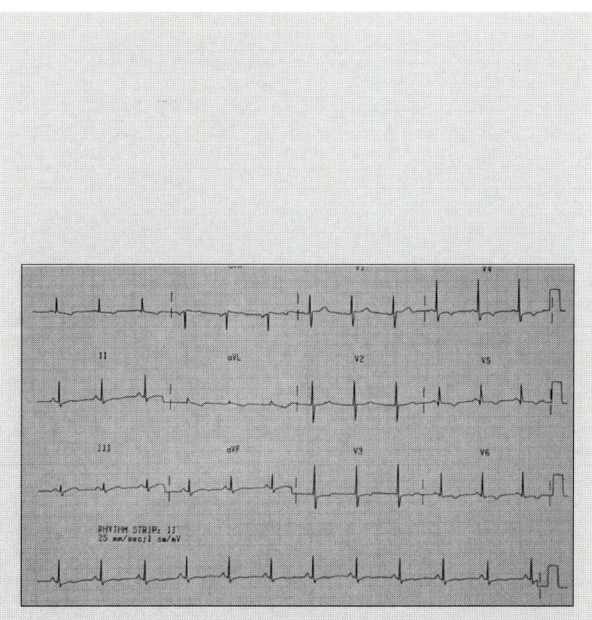

Figure 36 Same patient as in Figure 35 24 hours after the administration of streptokinase. The inferior leads look normal but the R wave in leads V1 and V2 has become more positive, probably indicating posterior infarction. The lateral T wave changes remain

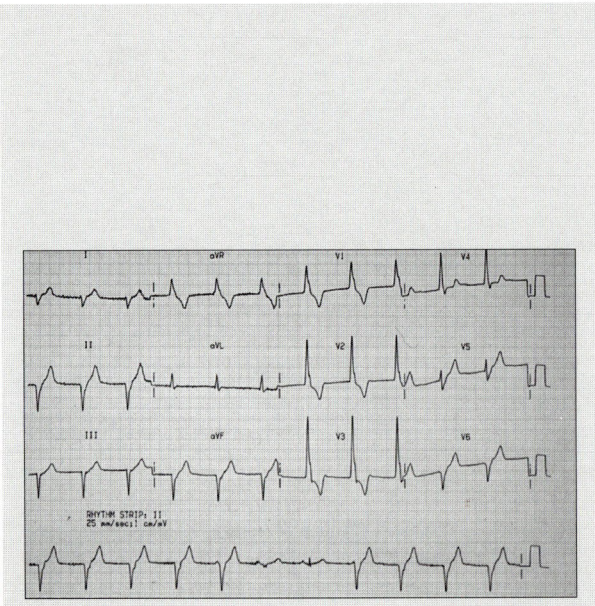

Figure 37 ECG from a patient with 2 hours of prolonged central chest pain. The rhythm is an idioventricular rhythm with no P wave before each QRS complex and with a right bundle branch block and left anterior hemiblock pattern. Two sinus beats are seen on the rhythm strip at the bottom. This arrhythmia was well tolerated

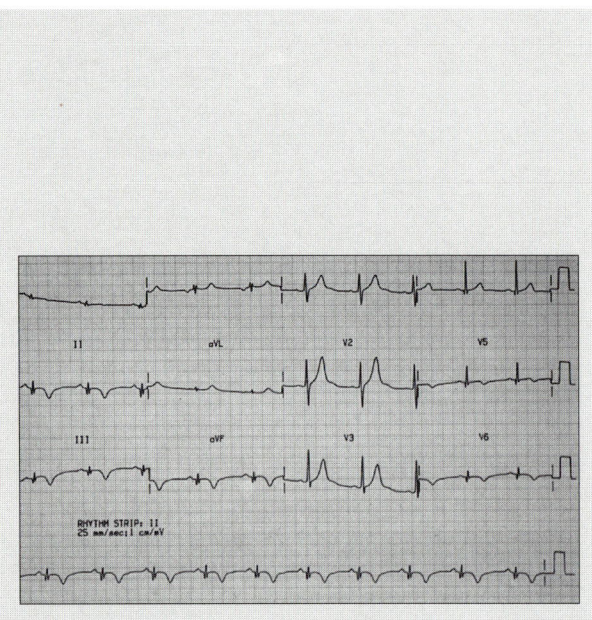

Figure 38 12-lead ECG from the same patient as in Figure 37 after streptokinase and reversion to sinus rhythm. Small Q waves and deep T wave inversion are seen in leads II, III, AVF, V5 and V6, indicating a small inferolateral infarction

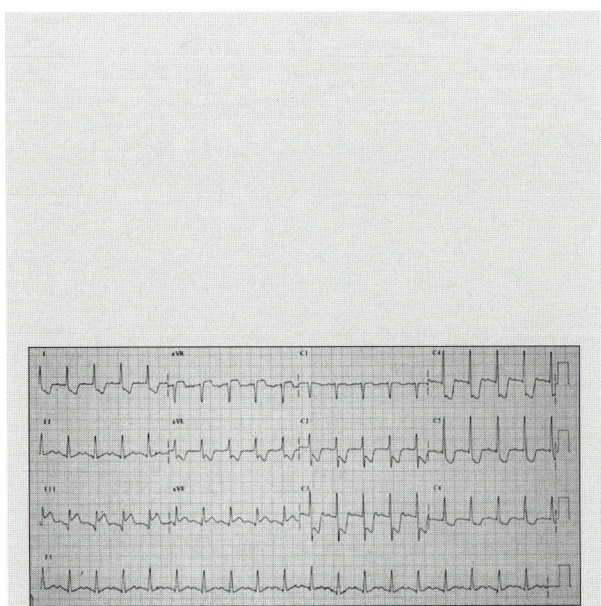

Figure 39 ECG from a patient presenting with an acute inferior infarction with ST elevation in leads III and AVF, but very impressive ST segment depression in leads I, AVL and V2–V6, all so-called reciprocal changes

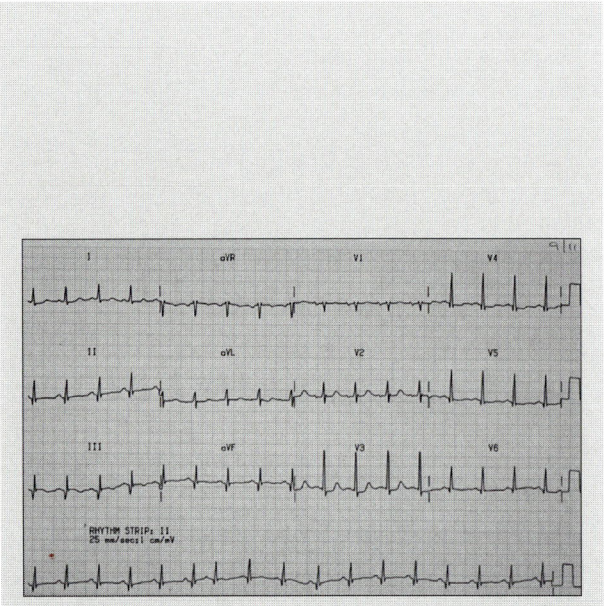

Figure 40 Same patient as in Figure 39 24 hours later having been given streptokinase. This ECG now shows small Q waves in leads II, III, AVF and V6 with well-preserved R waves and incomplete right bundle branch block. The latter is of no significance

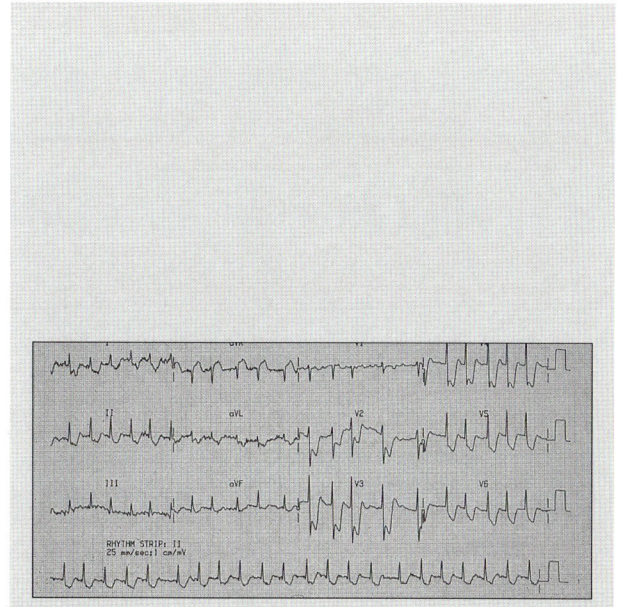

Figure 41 12-lead ECG from a patient presenting with 6 hours of prolonged ischemic chest pain. There is no ST segment elevation but there is profound (up to 10 mm) ST segment depression, particularly obvious in the anterior chest leads. The patient is in atrial fibrillation

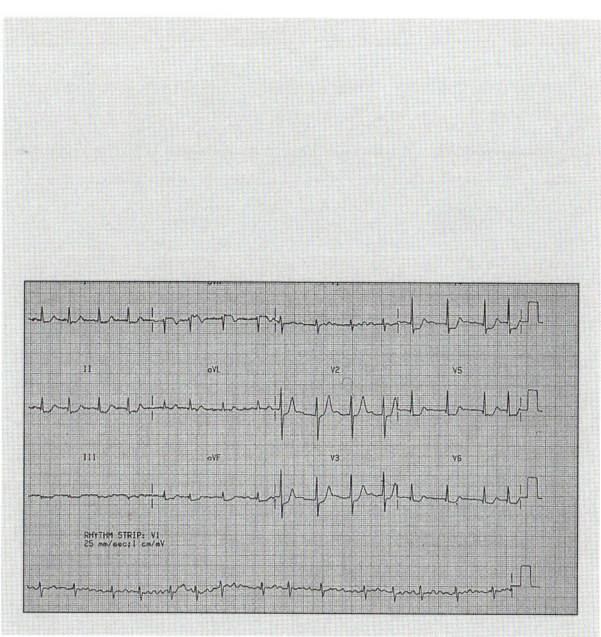

Figure 42 Same patient as in Figure 41 after administration of streptokinase. Atrial fibrillation persists but the ST segments have dramatically improved

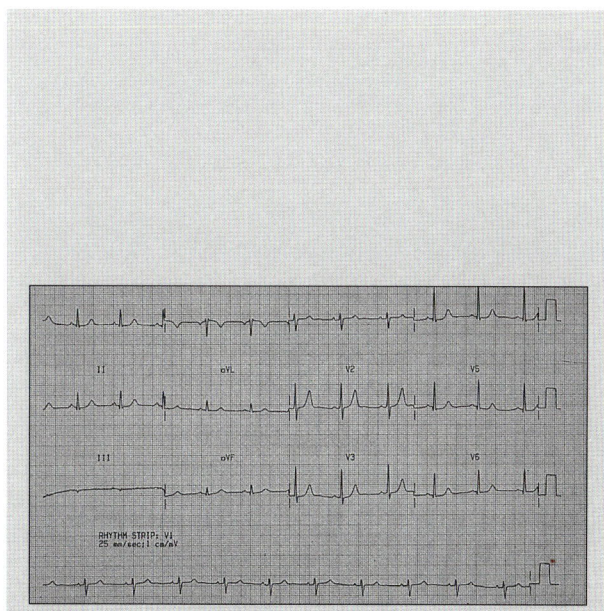

Figure 43 Same patient as in Figures 41 and 42 24 hours later having reverted to sinus rhythm. The ECG is normal, although the patient had a rise in total creatine phosphokinase and in the MB isoenzyme

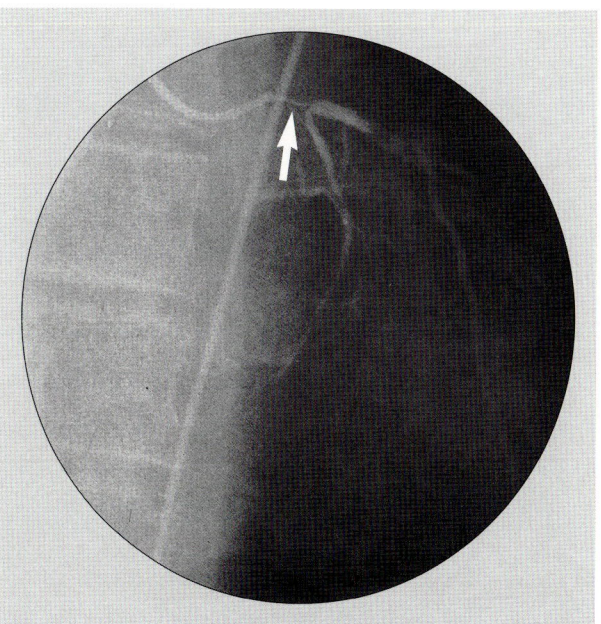

Figure 44 Coronary angiogram from the same patient as in Figures 41–43 showing extremely tight left main stem stenosis (arrowed) before the division of the left coronary into the circumflex and left anterior descending branches. The lesion is seen just as the ascending limb of the catheter crosses the left coronary artery

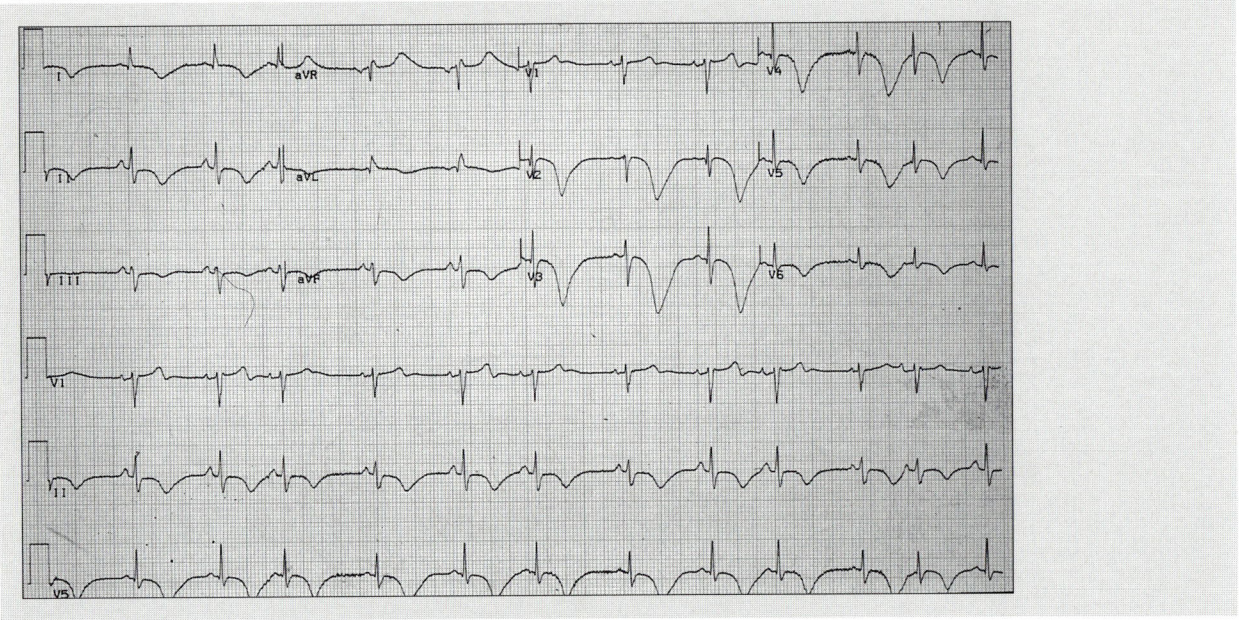

Figure 45 Anterior and inferior non-Q wave myocardial infarction with deep T wave inversion across the front of the chest and inferiorly but no Q waves. The patient had recurrent pain in hospital and was transferred for angiography

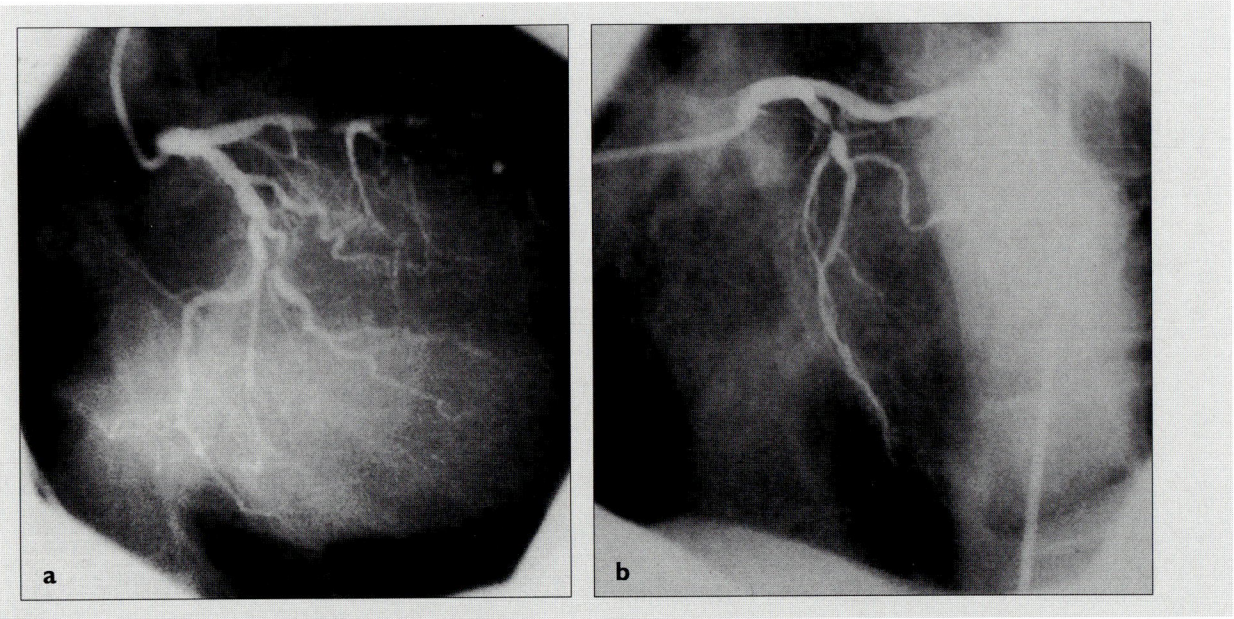

Figure 46 (a) Right anterior oblique and (b) left anterior oblique coronary angiograms from the same patient as in Figure 45. There is an exquisitely tight left anterior descending stenosis seen in both projections

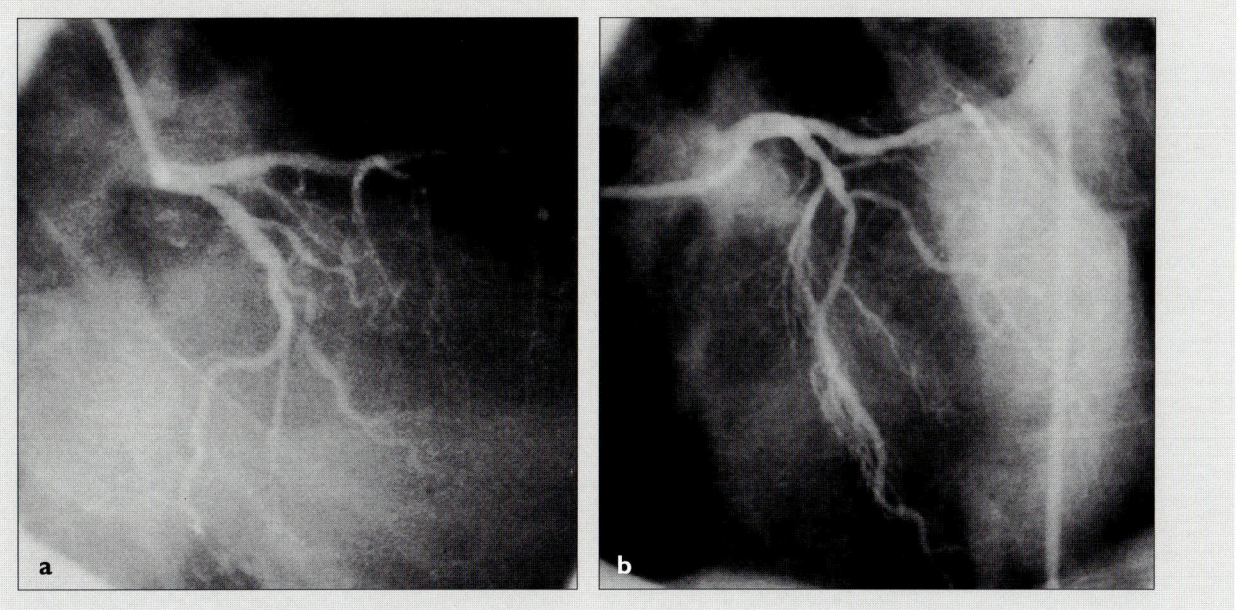

Figure 47 Same patient, same views as in Figures 45 and 46, after emergency coronary angioplasty for continuing pain. Note abolition of the stenosis

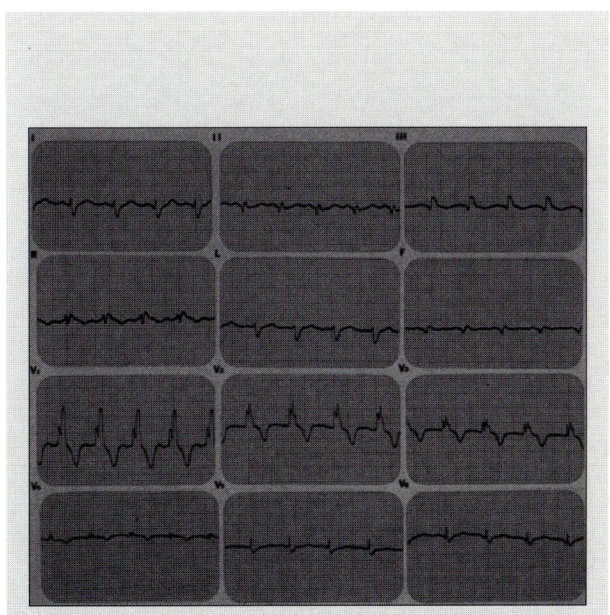

Figure 48 12-lead ECG showing inferior myocardial infarction and complete right bundle branch block

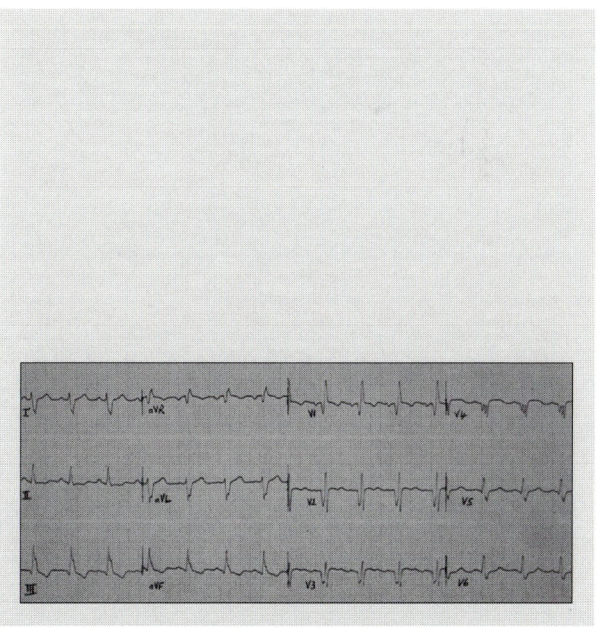

Figure 49 Anteroseptal myocardial infarction with Q waves anteriorly and right bundle branch block

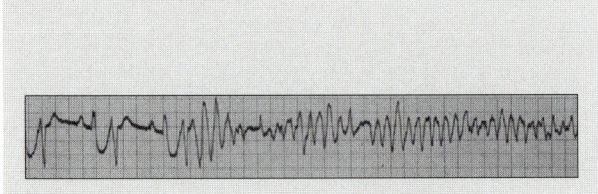

Figure 50 Rhythm strip from a patient with an acute myocardial infarction. Note the first three sinus beats are followed by an R-on-T ectopic, the third of which precipitates primary ventricular fibrillation, characterized by chaotic electrical activity

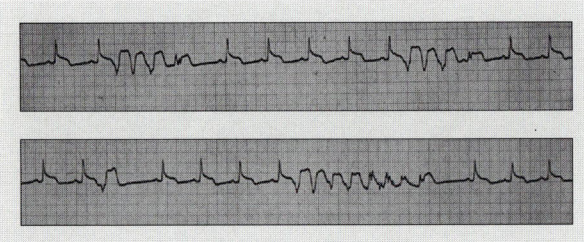

Figure 51 Rhythm strip showing ST segment elevation on the sinus beats with several bursts of non-sustained ventricular tachycardia

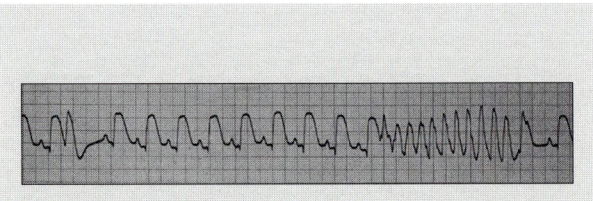

Figure 52 Rhythm strip showing very marked ST segment elevation in the sinus beats and one burst of rapid non-sustained ventricular tachycardia. This occurred during an infusion of streptokinase and is often called a reperfusion arrhythmia

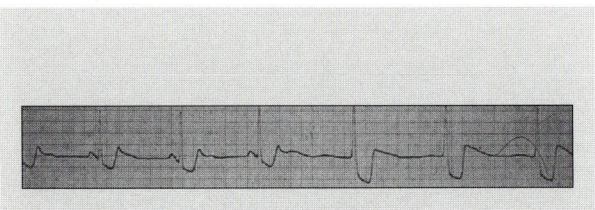

Figure 53 Rhythm strip from a patient with an inferior myocardial infarction showing sinus arrest with a narrow complex junctional escape rhythm. Note the sudden disappearance of the P waves after the third complete beat

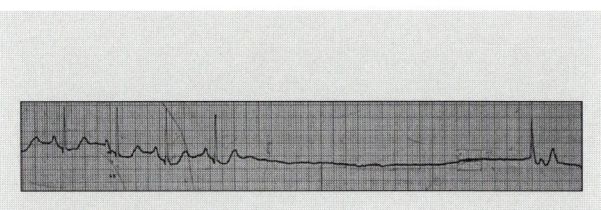

Figure 54 Rhythm strip from a patient with an inferior infarction showing sudden and severe sinus arrest. The 5-second pause is terminated by a junctional escape beat

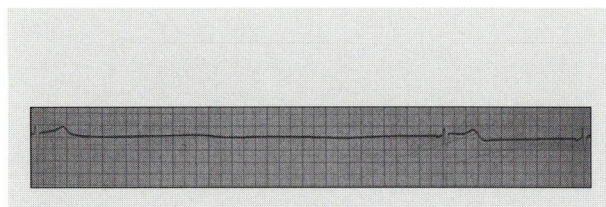

Figure 55 An even more extreme example of a sinus arrest after an inferior infarction with a pause of 7 seconds

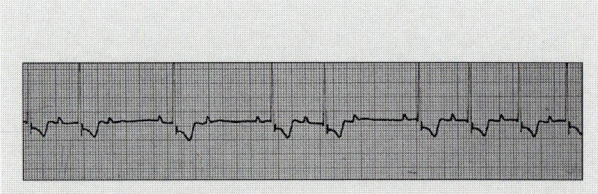

Figure 56 Rhythm strip from a patient with an inferior myocardial infarction showing atrioventricular Wenkebach phenomenon (Mobitz I) with prolongation of the PR interval before a QRS complex is dropped. Occasionally, as on this rhythm strip, 2:1 Wenkebach occurs. The site of block is usually in the atrioventricular node

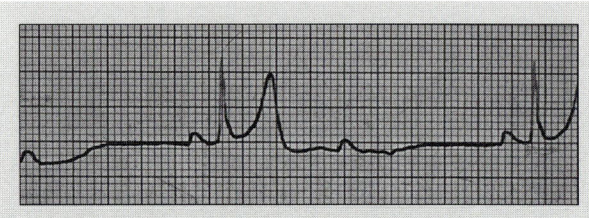

Figure 57 A rhythm strip showing another example of 2:1 heart block after inferior infarction

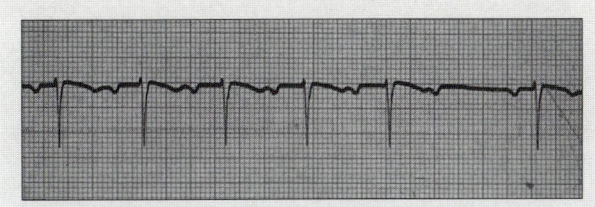

Figure 58 Another example of the Wenkebach phenomenon

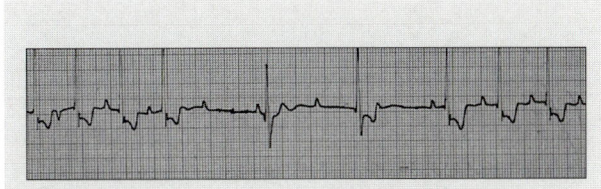

Figure 59 Rhythm strip from a patient with an anterior infarction showing Mobitz II, second-degree heart block where the PR interval does not prolong before a QRS complex is dropped. The first QRS complex after the block is probably an escape beat and the subsequent beat may be a sinus beat conducted with an extremely long PR interval. The site of block is usually infranodal

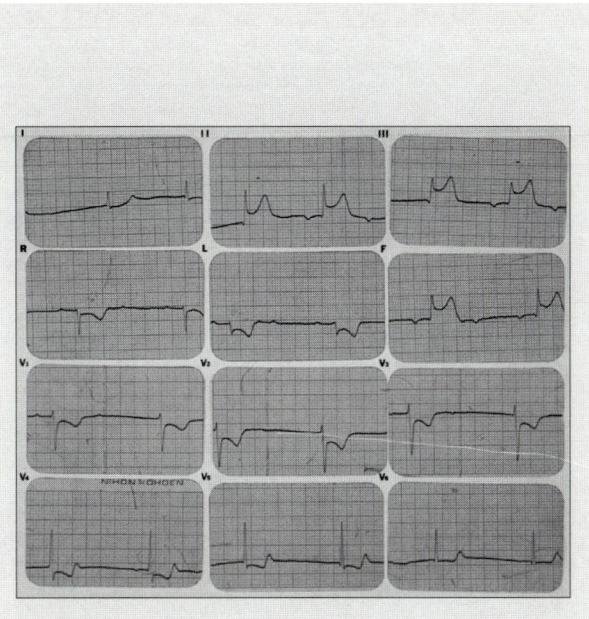

Figure 60 12-lead ECG showing an acute inferior myocardial infarction with T wave inversion anteriorly and complete atrioventricular block with a narrow QRS escape complex. This is typical of inferior infarction and the block is usually temporary

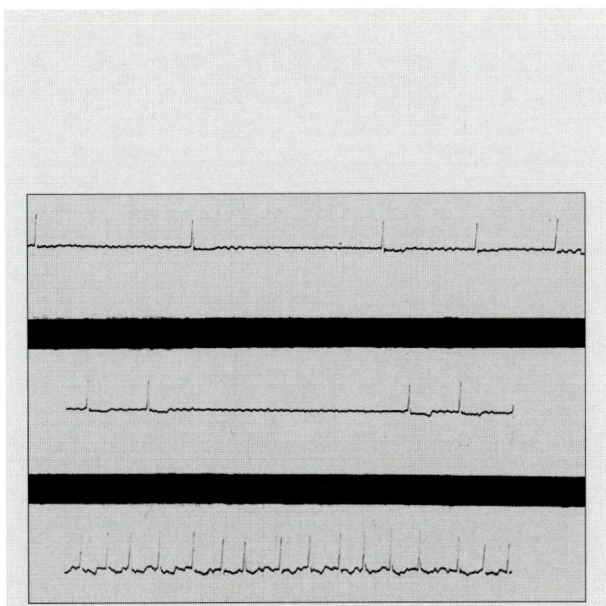

Figure 61 Rhythm strip from a patient with an inferior myocardial infarction showing atrial fibrillation and ventricular standstill (upper and middle panels). Normal conduction is resumed in the lower panel

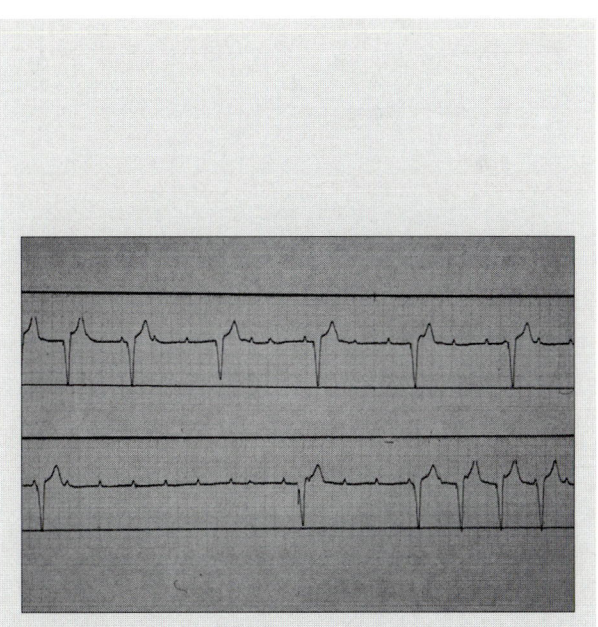

Figure 62 Rhythm strip showing a patient with an anterior myocardial infarction and a temporary pacemaker *in situ*. Note that, when the pacemaker is turned down, there is no spontaneous ventricular rhythm and the patient is pacing dependent. Only spontaneous P wave activity is seen

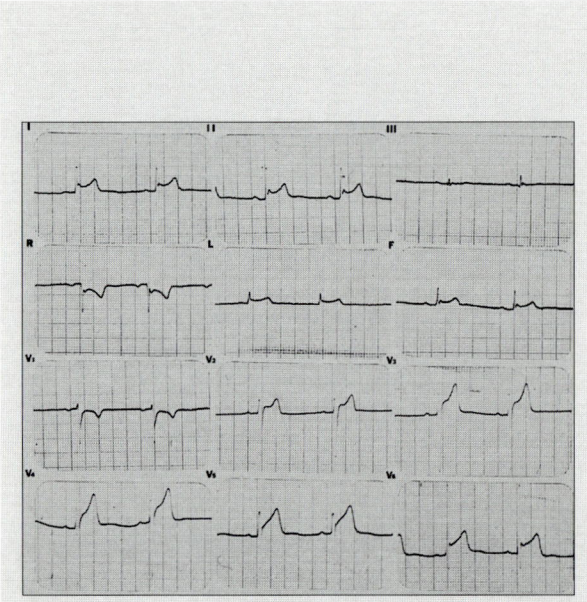

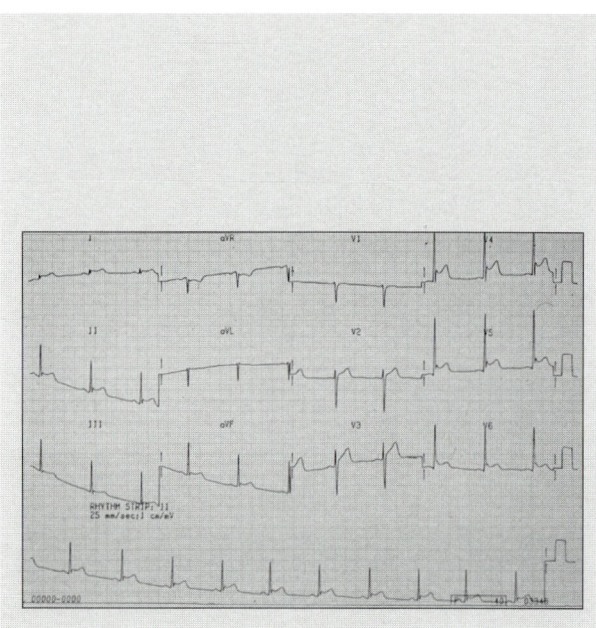

Figure 63 12-lead ECG in a patient presenting with chest pain. This is acute pericarditis and can sometimes be confused with acute myocardial infarction. The shape of the elevated ST segments is concave upwards and all the leads of the electrocardiogram are involved. The history plus the ECG appearances should make differentiation from acute myocardial infarction reasonably straightforward

Figure 64 12-lead electrocardiogram from African patient presenting with chest pain, initially thought to be showing signs of acute myocardial infarction. The high 'J' point and the high takeoff ST segments are often seen in Africans as a normal finding and are sometimes called a 'racial variant'. This should be borne in mind if thrombolytic therapy is to be considered

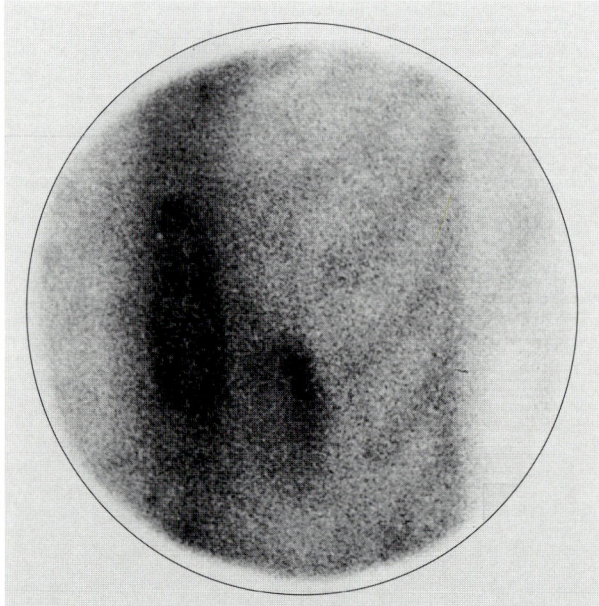

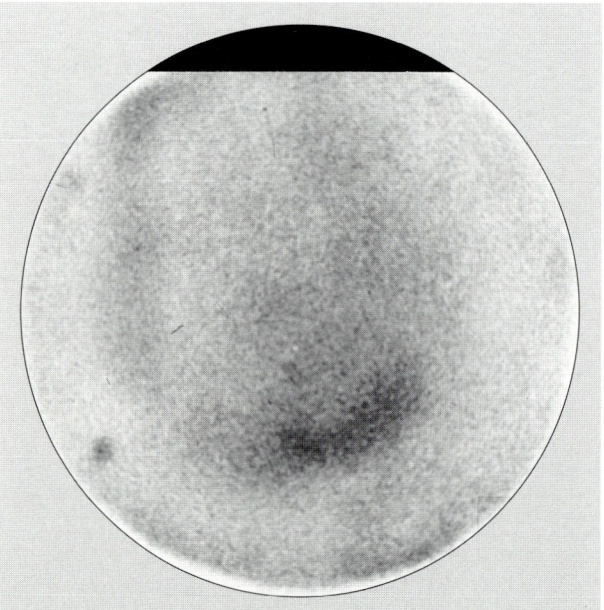

Figure 65 ⁹⁹ᵐTc-labelled stannous pyrophosphate infarct scan. The agent is taken up by bones so the sternum and rib cage are well seen. Between the bony structures, however, there is dense uptake in the region of the myocardium, which is most concentrated in the anterolateral wall in this projection. The scan was taken 24 hours after a patient presented with ECG changes of an anterolateral myocardial infarction. This is a so-called 'hot-spot' scan

Figure 66 Left anterior oblique pyrophosphate scan in a patient with a posterior and apical infarction. The sternum is seen to the left-hand side of the picture and the crescent-shaped uptake is seen in the posterior and apical regions of the myocardium

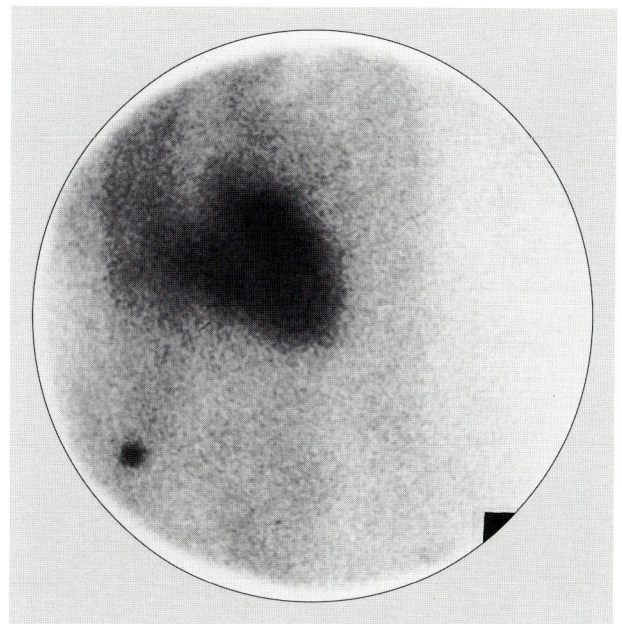

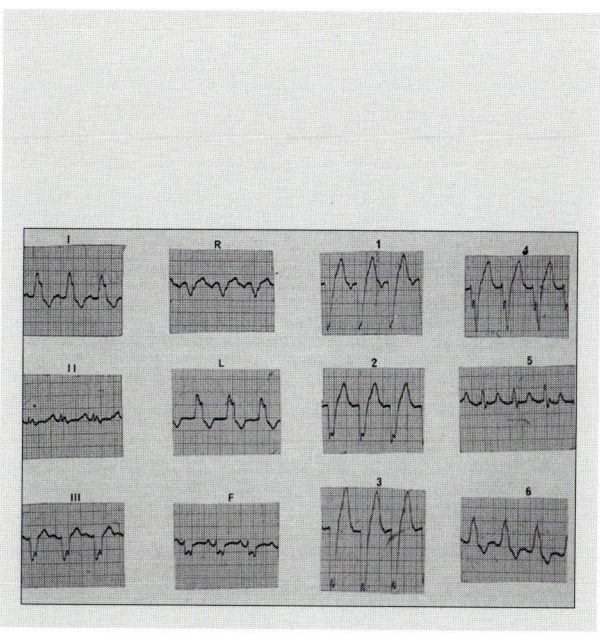

Figure 67 Anteroposterior scan showing extremely dense uptake of pyrophosphate in the region of the myocardium. This patient sustained a massive infarct with pulmonary edema. Uptake is seen in the anterior wall, the apex and the inferior wall and is very dense

Figure 68 12-lead ECG showing complete left bundle branch block in a patient presenting with prolonged chest pain. The left bundle branch block disguises the changes of anterior infarction but the patient sustained an enzyme rise

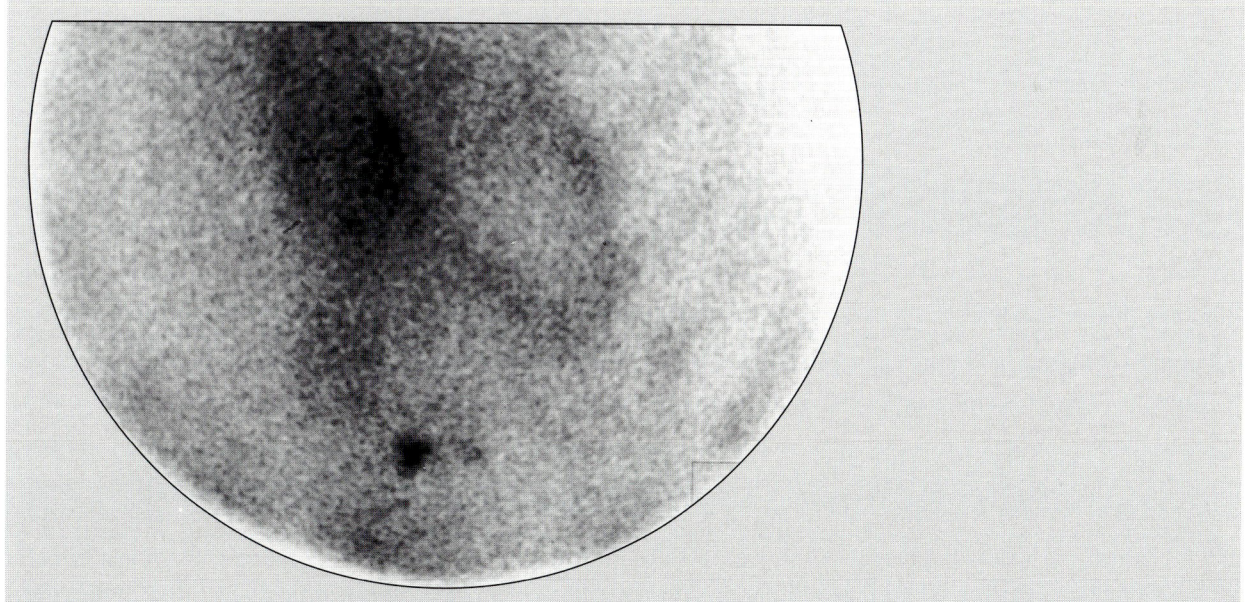

Figure 69 Anteroposterior pyrophosphate scan from the same patient as in Figure 68. A rim of technetium pyrophosphate is seen around the periphery of the infarct but not in the center. This is sometimes called a 'doughnut' scan and it is postulated that the absence of flow to the center of the infarct is responsible for the failure of delivery of the isotope to that region and, therefore, its uptake is only on the edges. Such appearances may imply an adverse prognosis and are usually only seen in large infarcts

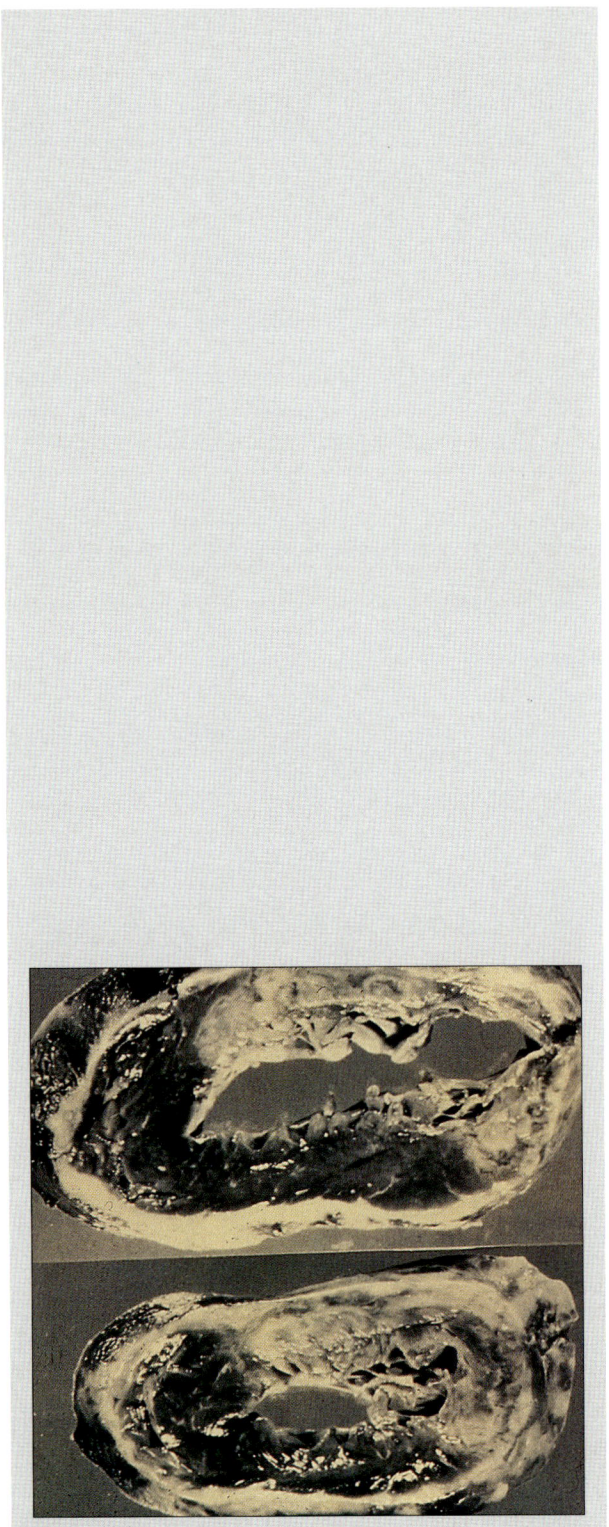

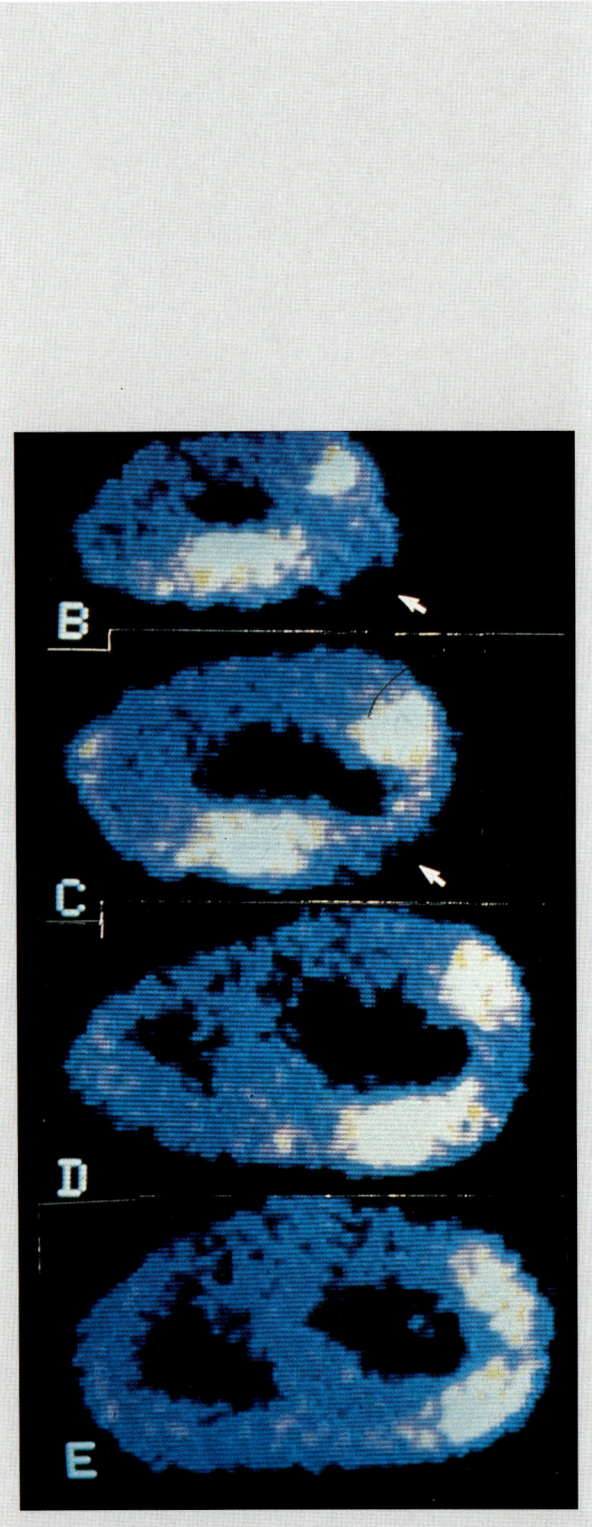

Figure 70 Two sections from a postmortem heart stained for succinic dehydrogenase. The pale areas are the areas of necrosis with enzyme loss. The right ventricle is seen on the left side. Note that the interventricular septum is intact

Figure 71 Same postmortem heart as in Figure 70 imaged scintigraphically with a gamma camera, as the patient had been injected with [111In]anti-myosin prior to his demise. The dense areas of [111In]anti-myosin uptake are seen as white on these sections and the blue areas represent residual indium in the intramyocardial circulation but without active uptake. The areas of dense white uptake correspond partially to the areas of enzyme loss in Figure 70. Note that there is some patchy right ventricular uptake as well but no uptake in the intraventricular septum

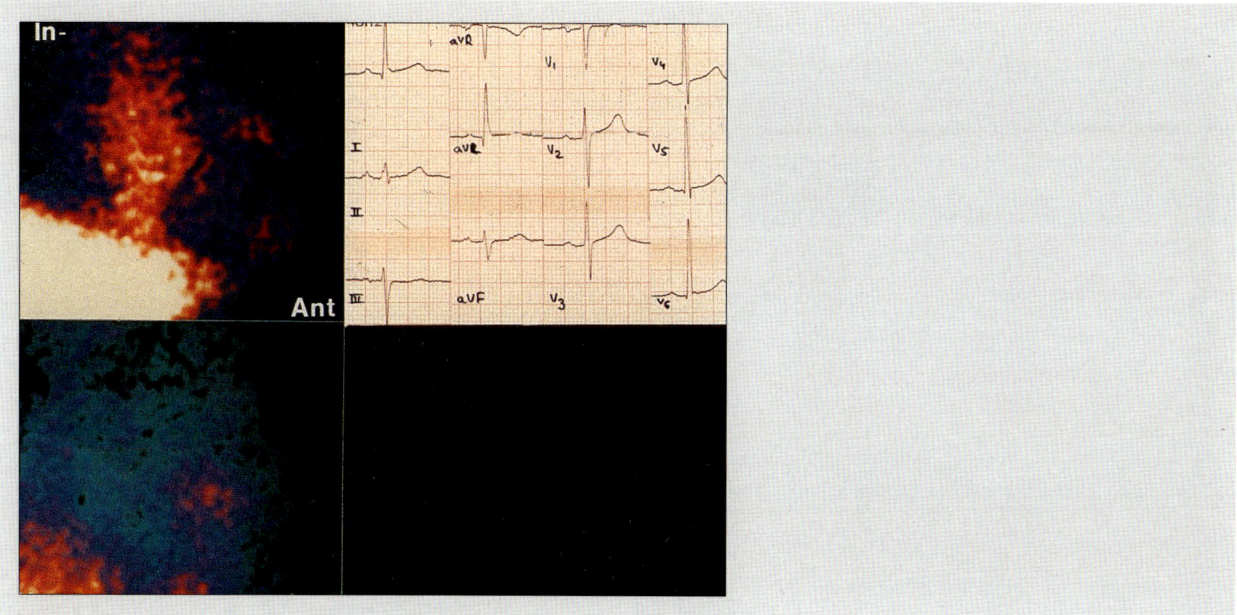

Figure 72 Positive [¹¹¹In]anti-myosin scan in a patient with a normal ECG. The anteroposterior and left anterior oblique scans are shown in the upper and lower left panels and the ECG on the top right. The technique is more sensitive than an ECG for detecting myocardial necrosis. Note that, unlike pyrophosphate, [¹¹¹In]anti-myosin does not demonstrate the bony structures

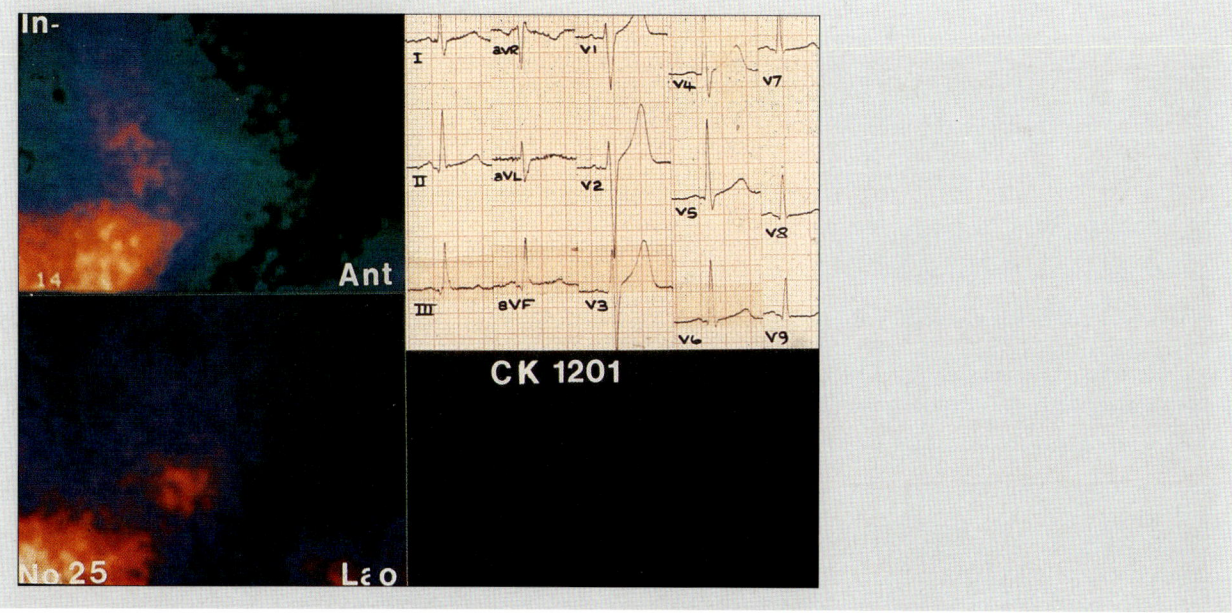

Figure 73 Another example of uptake of [¹¹¹In]anti-myosin in both anteroposterior and left anterior oblique views in the presence of a normal ECG but with a raised creatine kinase level

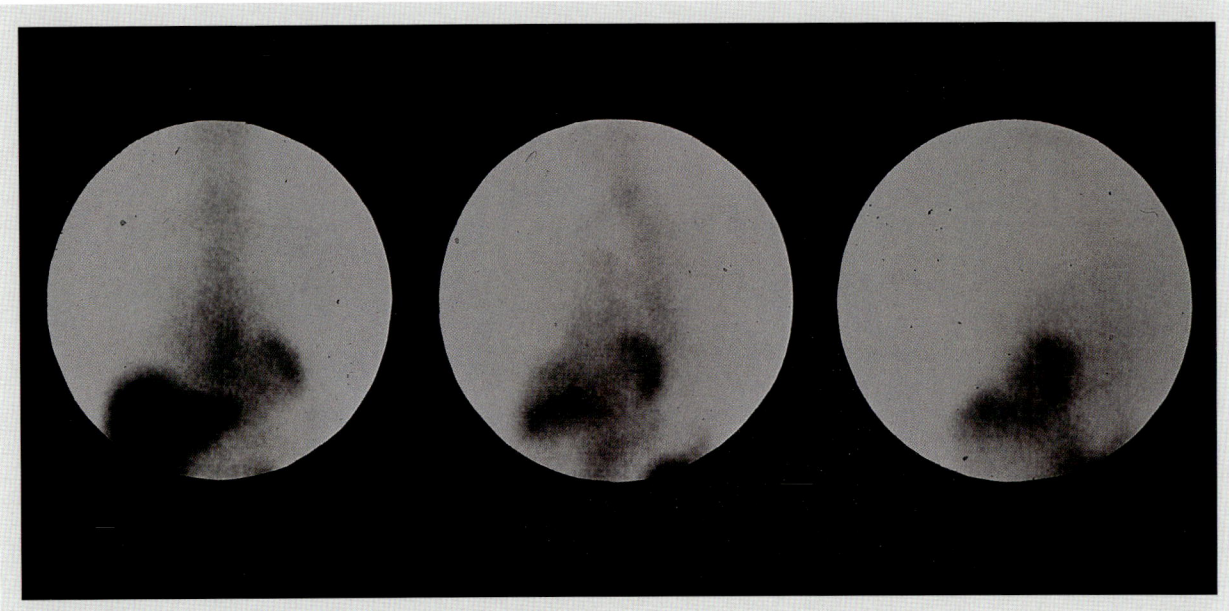

Figure 74 Anterior (left), left anterior oblique (middle) and left lateral (right hand) anti-myosin scans 48 hours after acute infarction. Dense uptake is seen anterolaterally and posterolaterally and in the splanchnic viscera

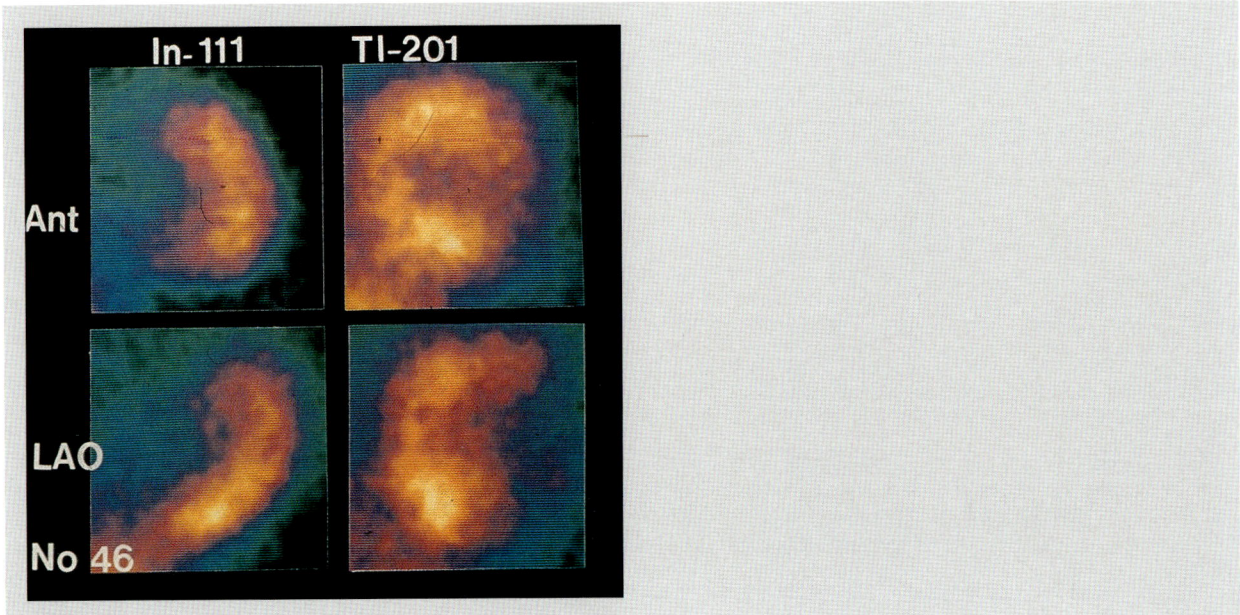

Figure 75 Combined [¹¹¹In] anti-myosin and thallium-201 images in patient with myocardial infarction. Thallium only accumulates in areas of normal perfusion and is not actively taken up by infarcted muscle. Note that the areas of indium uptake are matched by areas of deficient thallium uptake

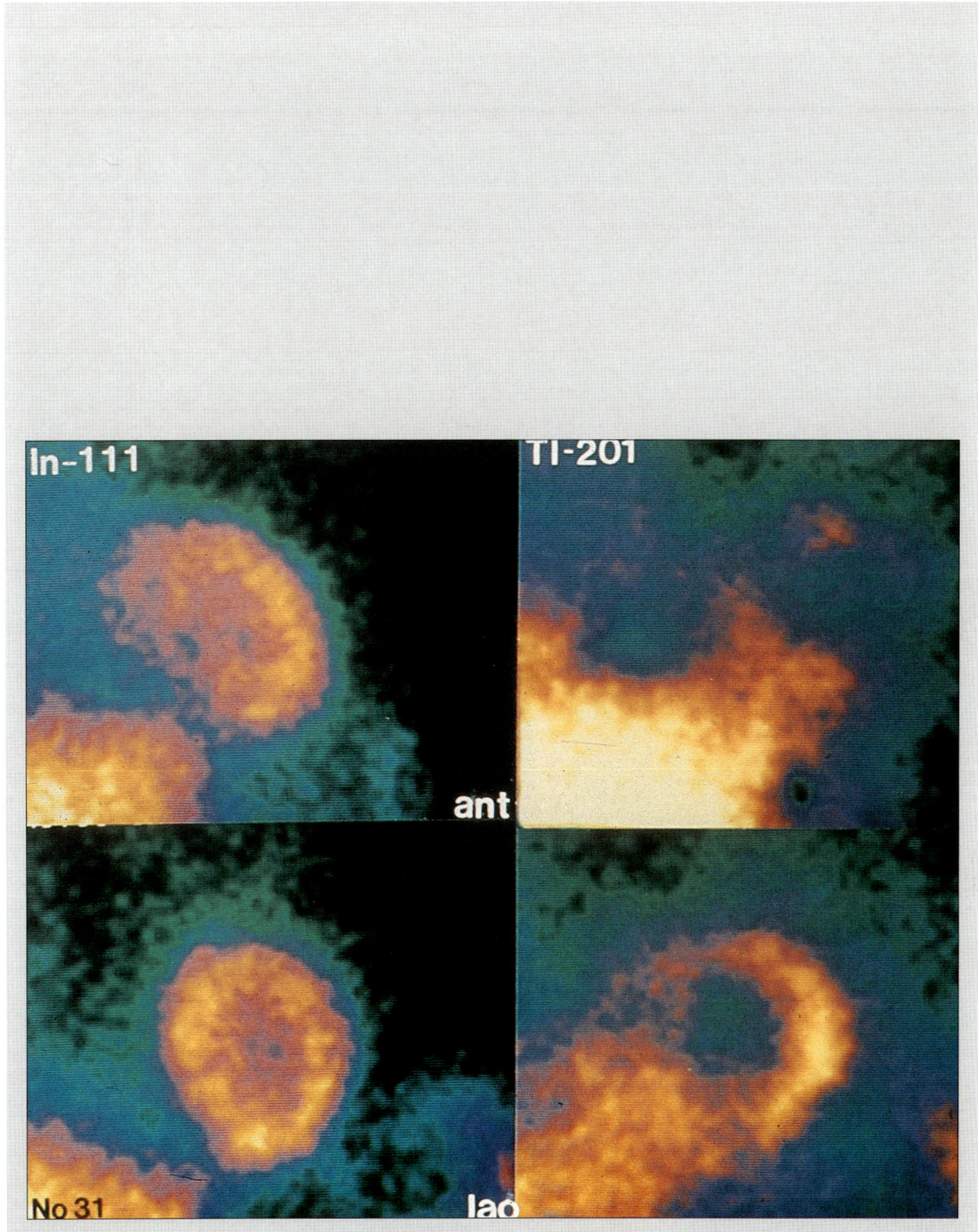

Figure 76 Another example of intense [¹¹¹In]anti-myosin uptake in anterior and left anterior oblique projections with extensive thallium defects in the anterior projection, although the bottom two panels suggest that there is both indium uptake and thallium uptake in the posterior wall. This may indicate areas of necrosis interspersed with areas of viable muscle

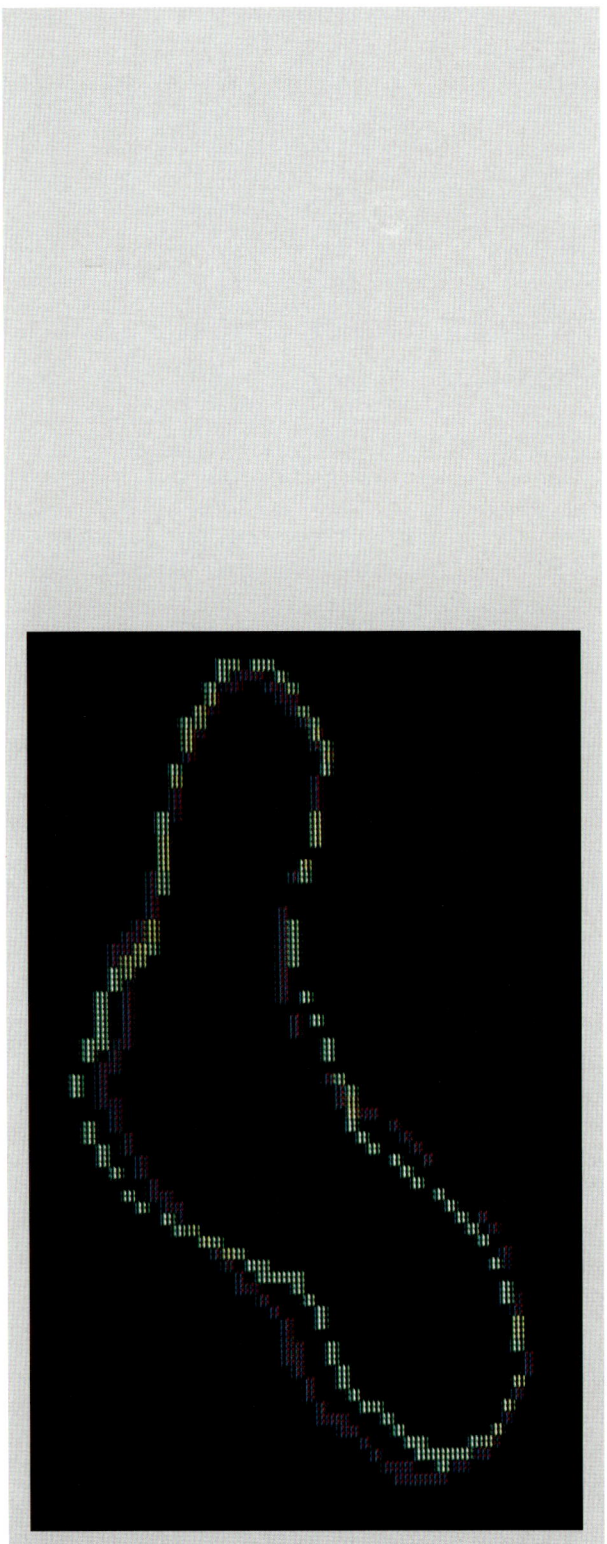

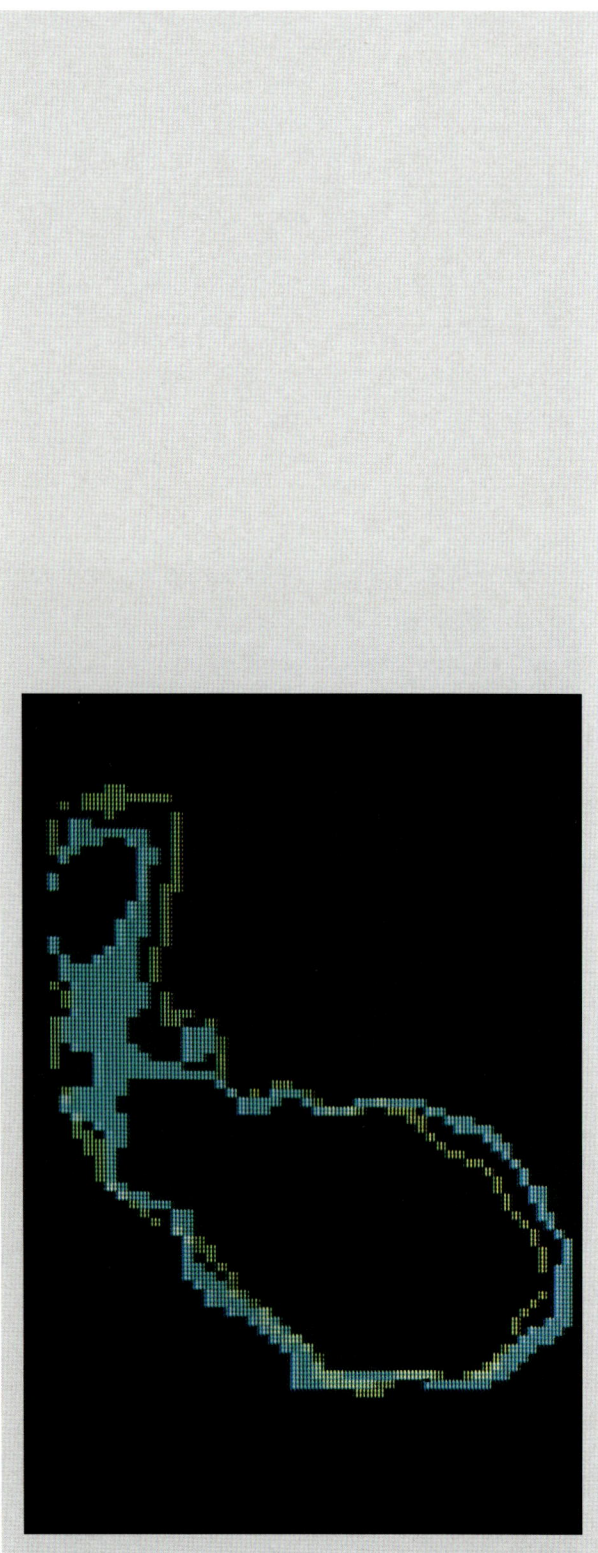

Figure 77 Image of end-systolic perimeter in blue, end-diastolic perimeter in purple from a first-pass radionuclide angiogram from a patient who sustained an anterior myocardial infarction. Note that in the anterior wall the two perimeters are virtually superimposed, whereas in the inferior wall and in the anterobasal segment the perimeters are separated and their positions at end-diastole and end-systole are seen. The superimposition of the two perimeters indicates akinesis

Figure 78 Same format in a patient with an extensive inferior infarction where the end-systolic perimeter is shown in yellow and the end-diastolic in blue. Note that the two perimeters are superimposed in the inferior wall but show separation in the anterior wall. This is a large inferior myocardial infarction

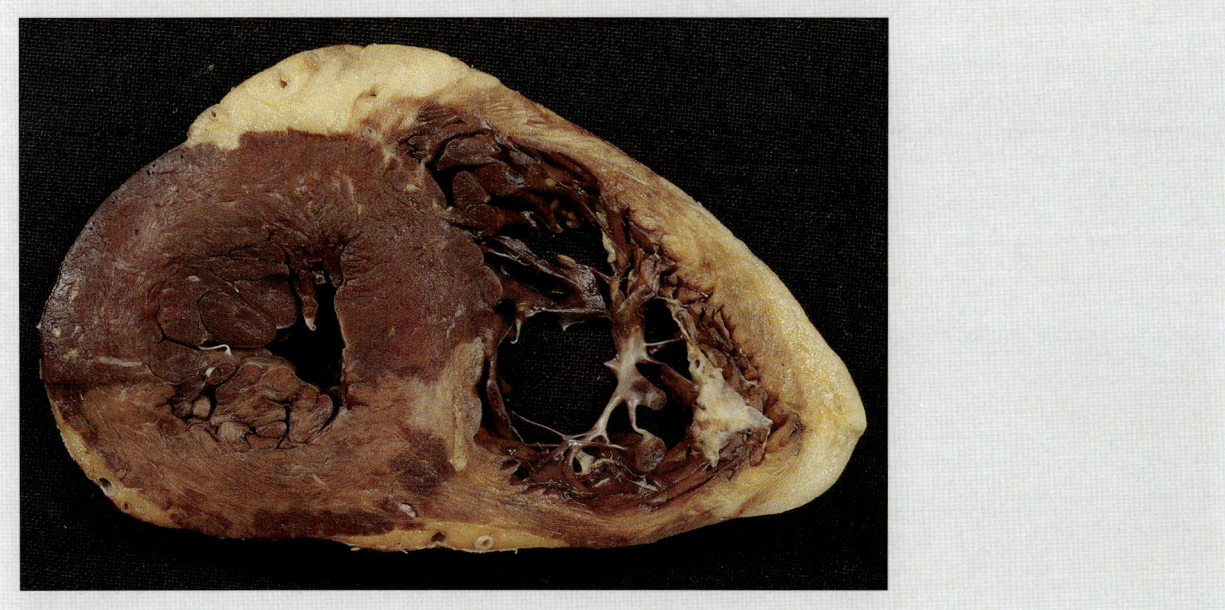

Figure 79 Cross-section of postmortem heart stained for succinic dehydrogenase. This mitochondrial enzyme stains blue in normal myocardium and pale in areas that show necrosis and loss of enzyme. Note the marked decrease of enzyme in the posterior wall and the whole of the right ventricle, indicating a significant right ventricular infarction associated with posterior infarction of the left ventricle

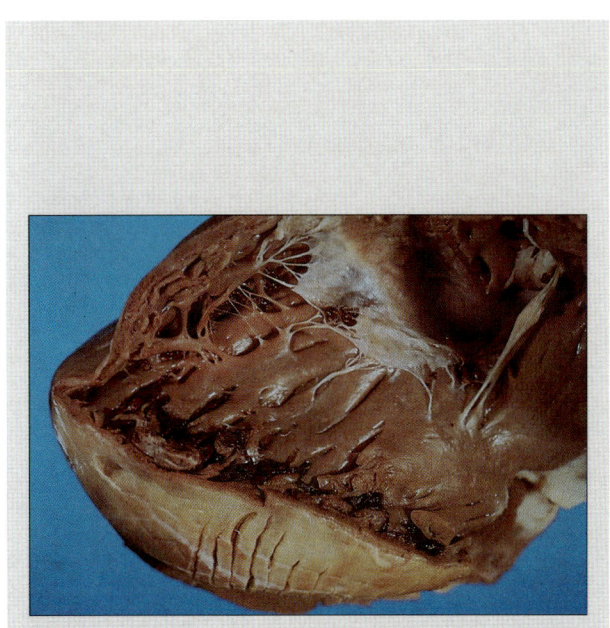

Figure 80 Thrombus in the right ventricle. This is an unusual complication

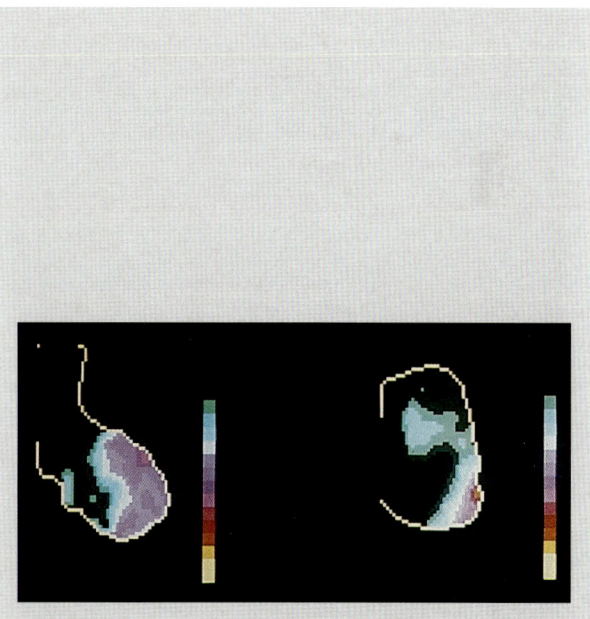

Figure 81 Regional ejection fraction images from the left and right ventricles in a patient with an inferior myocardial infarction. The left ventricular ejection fraction (39%) is moderately reduced and there is poor regional function of the left ventricle. The right ventricular ejection fraction is markedly reduced at 19%. The color bar indicates good regional function as yellow and red, decreasing through purple to green and black, the latter two colors indicating virtually absent regional function. (Reprinted with permission from *British Heart Journal*, 1987, **50**, 101–9)

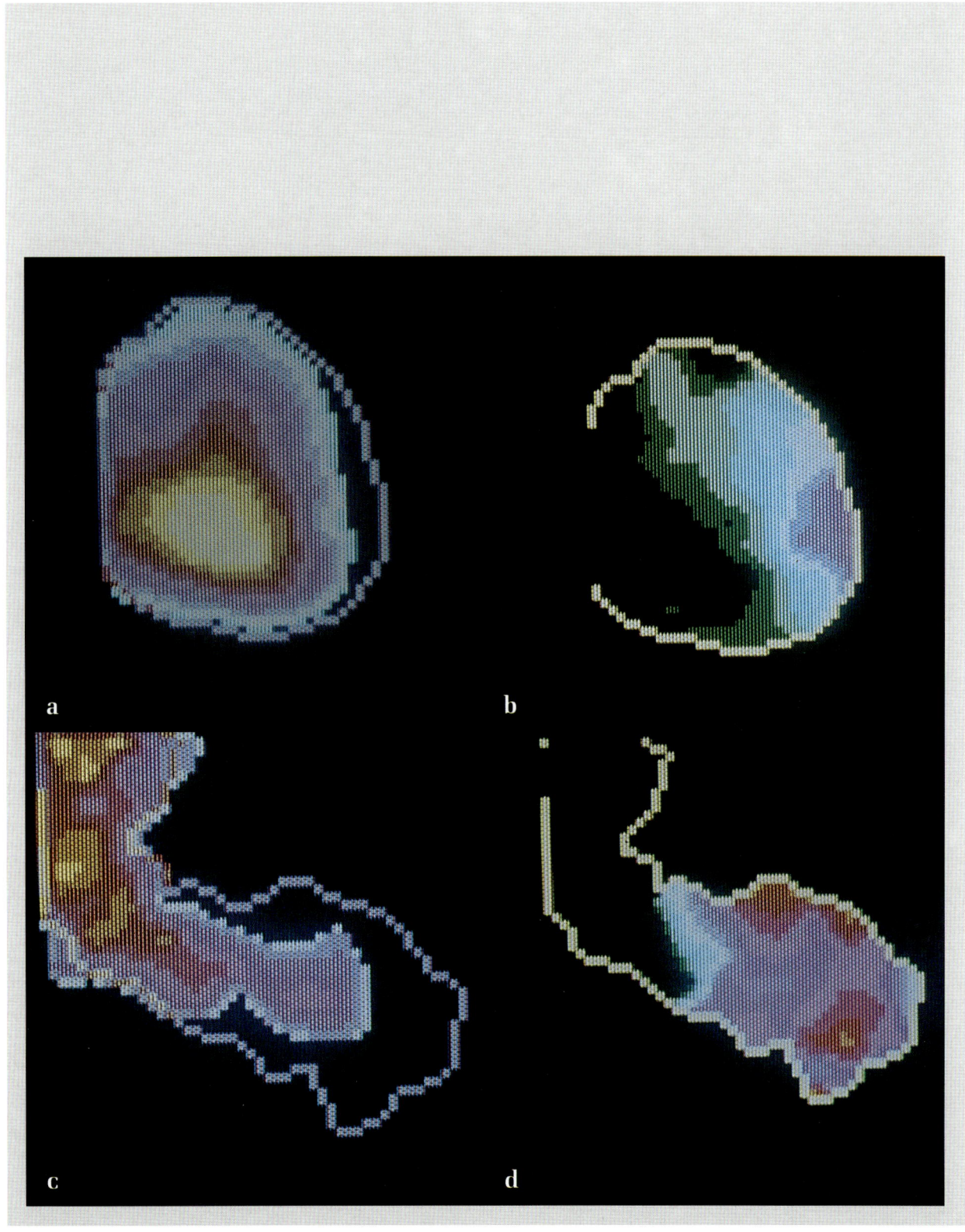

Figure 82 End-systolic images with end-diastolic perimeter superimposed for right and left ventricles (a and c, respectively) and regional ejection fraction images of right and left ventricles (b and d, respectively). Note that left ventri-cular function in this patient with a minor inferior infarction remains normal, whereas the right ventricle is grossly dilated and regional right ventricular function is globally poor

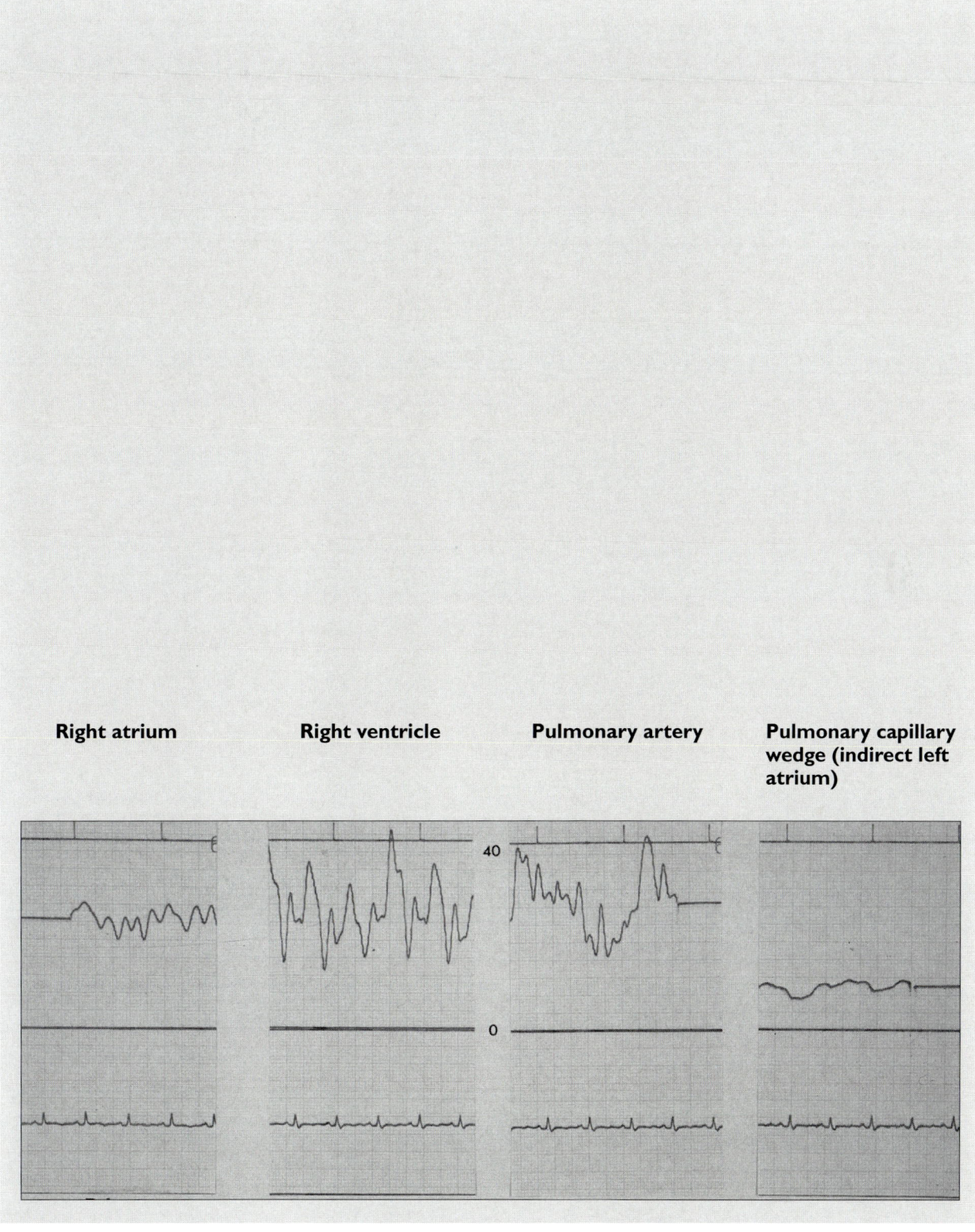

Right atrium　　**Right ventricle**　　**Pulmonary artery**　　**Pulmonary capillary wedge (indirect left atrium)**

Figure 83 Right-sided pressure traces from a patient with right ventricular infarction indicating, elevated right atrial and right ventricular pressures. The mean right atrial pressure is 24 mmHg, as is the right ventricular end-diastolic pressure. The mean wedge (PAW) is between 8 and 12 mmHg which is normal. It is wrong to give diuretics in this situation as the right ventricle needs a high filling pressure to drive it, in the presence of infarction

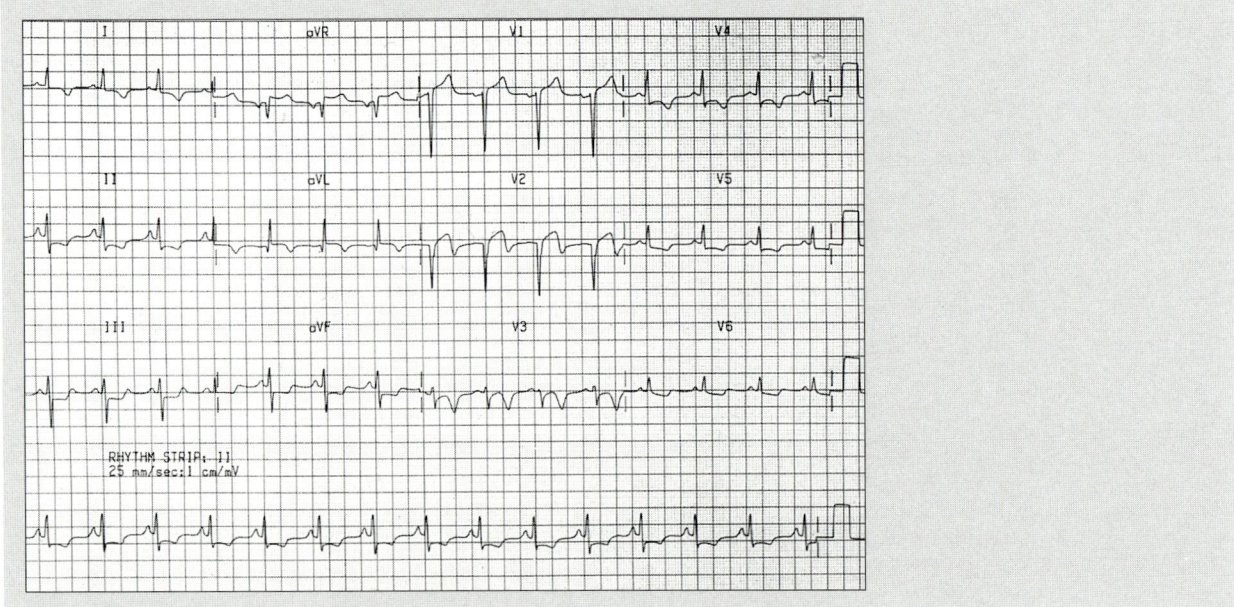

Figure 84 First stage of a 12-lead exercise test in a patient with an anterior infarction showing Q waves in VI and V2 and T wave inversion from VI to V3. At this early level of exercise, there is already some ST segment depression in leads II, III, AVF, V5 and V6 but with no pain

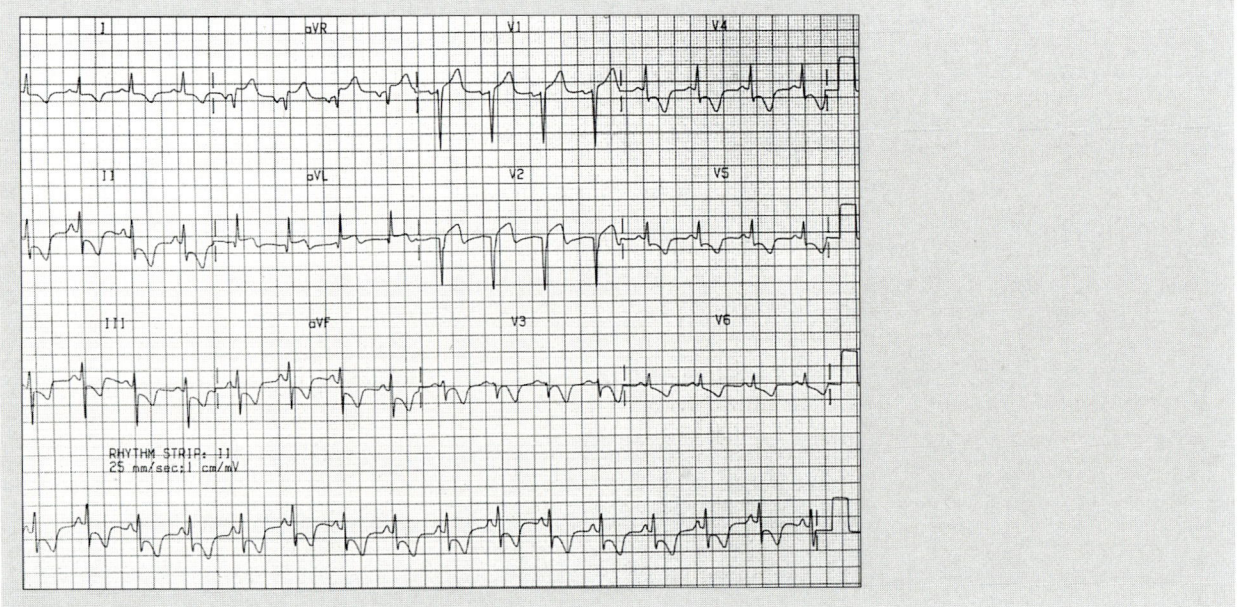

Figure 85 The end of stage two of the exercise protocol: there is now gross ST segment depression and T wave inversion in the inferior and lateral leads, which approaches 5 mmHg in lead II. The patient complained of mild chest pain

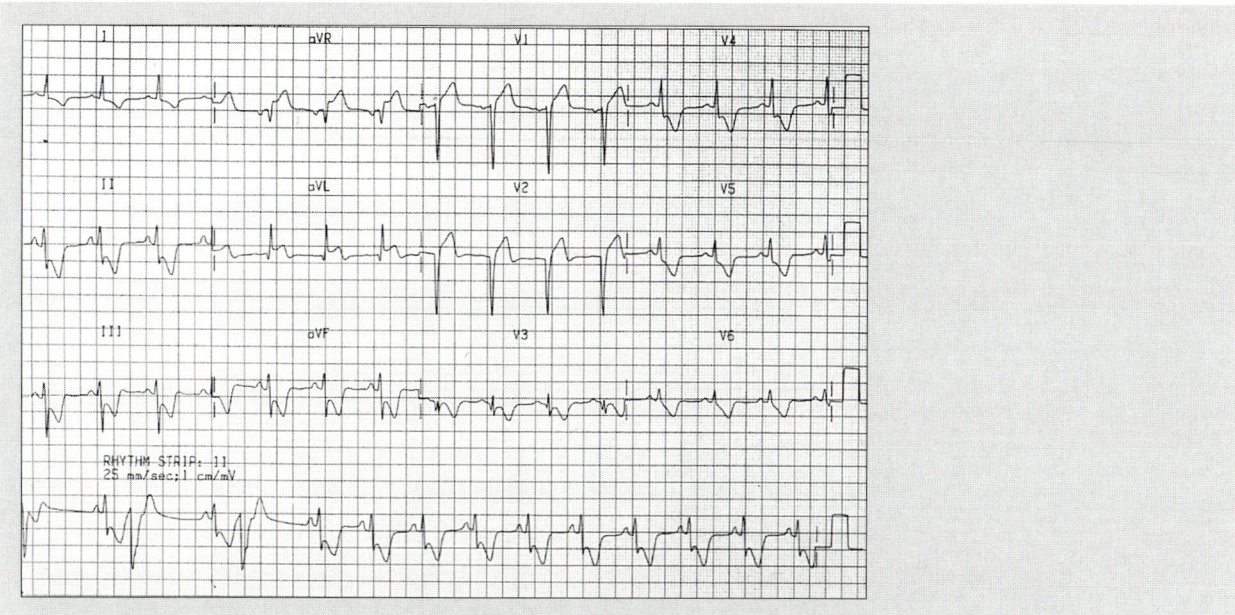

Figure 86 Same patient as in Figure 85 5 min into the recovery period showing persistent ST segment depression in the inferior and lateral leads, in addition to the anterior infarction changes. Also, the rhythm strip shows some ventricular bigeminy. The patient was subsequently found to have an occluded left anterior descending stenosis and a subtotal occlusion of the proximal right coronary artery, for which surgery was carried out

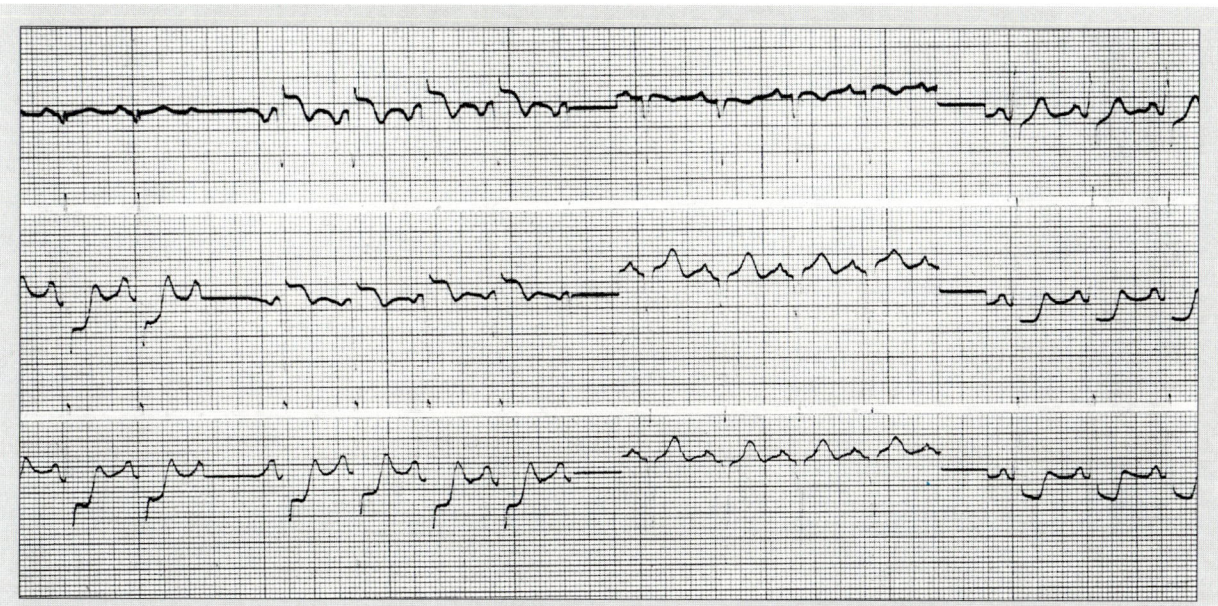

Figure 87 Submaximal pre-discharge exercise test in a patient who had sustained a small non-Q wave inferior infarction and whose resting ECG had returned to normal. Even at this relatively low heart rate, there is obvious planar ST segment depression in leads II, III, AVF and V5 and down-sloping in V6. This was unaccompanied by pain but angiography was undertaken and the patient underwent coronary angioplasty to the right coronary artery

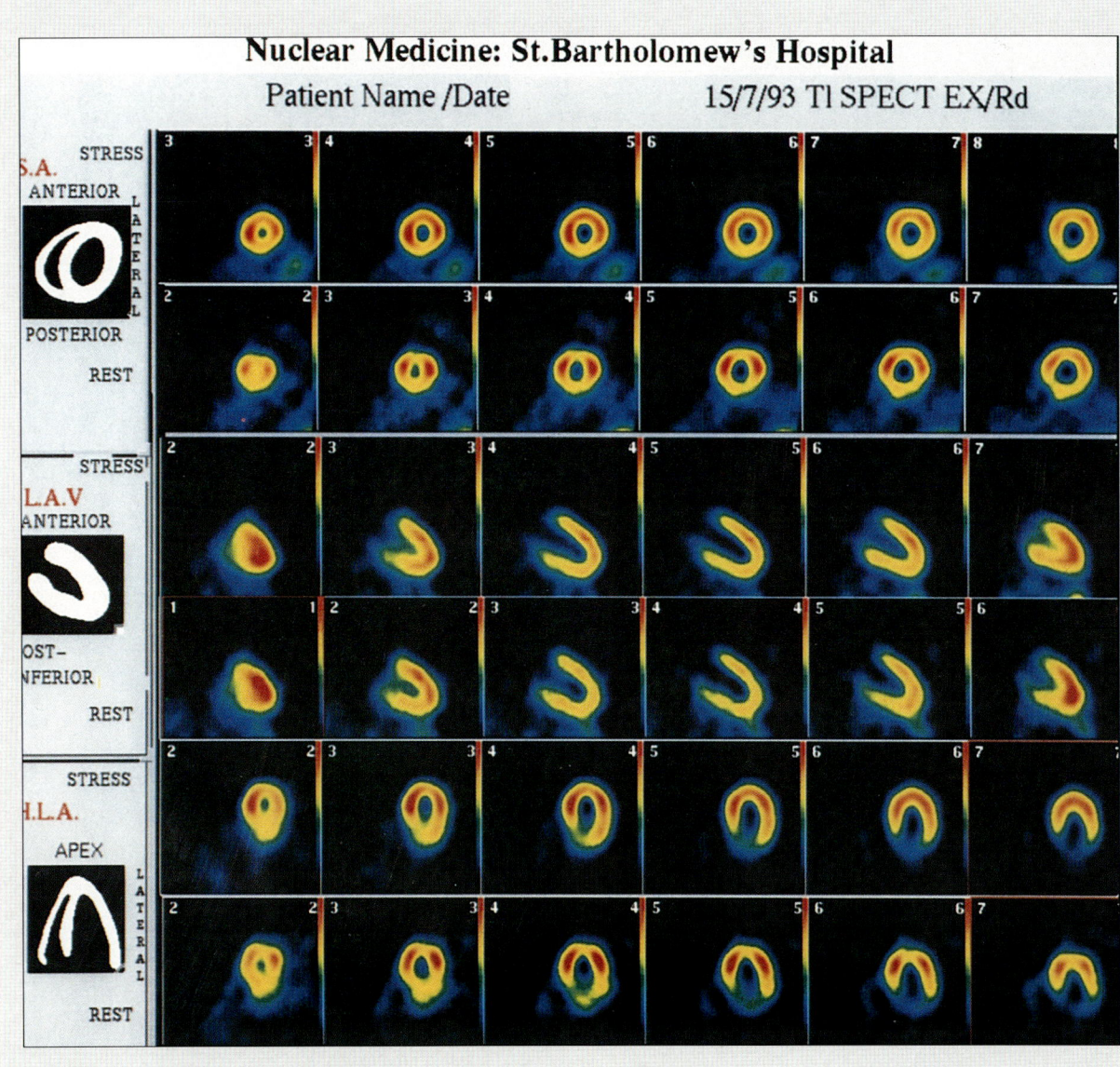

Figure 88 Normal thallium tomograms at exercise and redistribution in the short axis (upper two panels), vertical long axis (middle two panels), and horizontal long axis (lower two panels). Each pair of images in each axis allows the comparison of myocardial perfusion under stress and again at rest. This normal example is for reference purposes

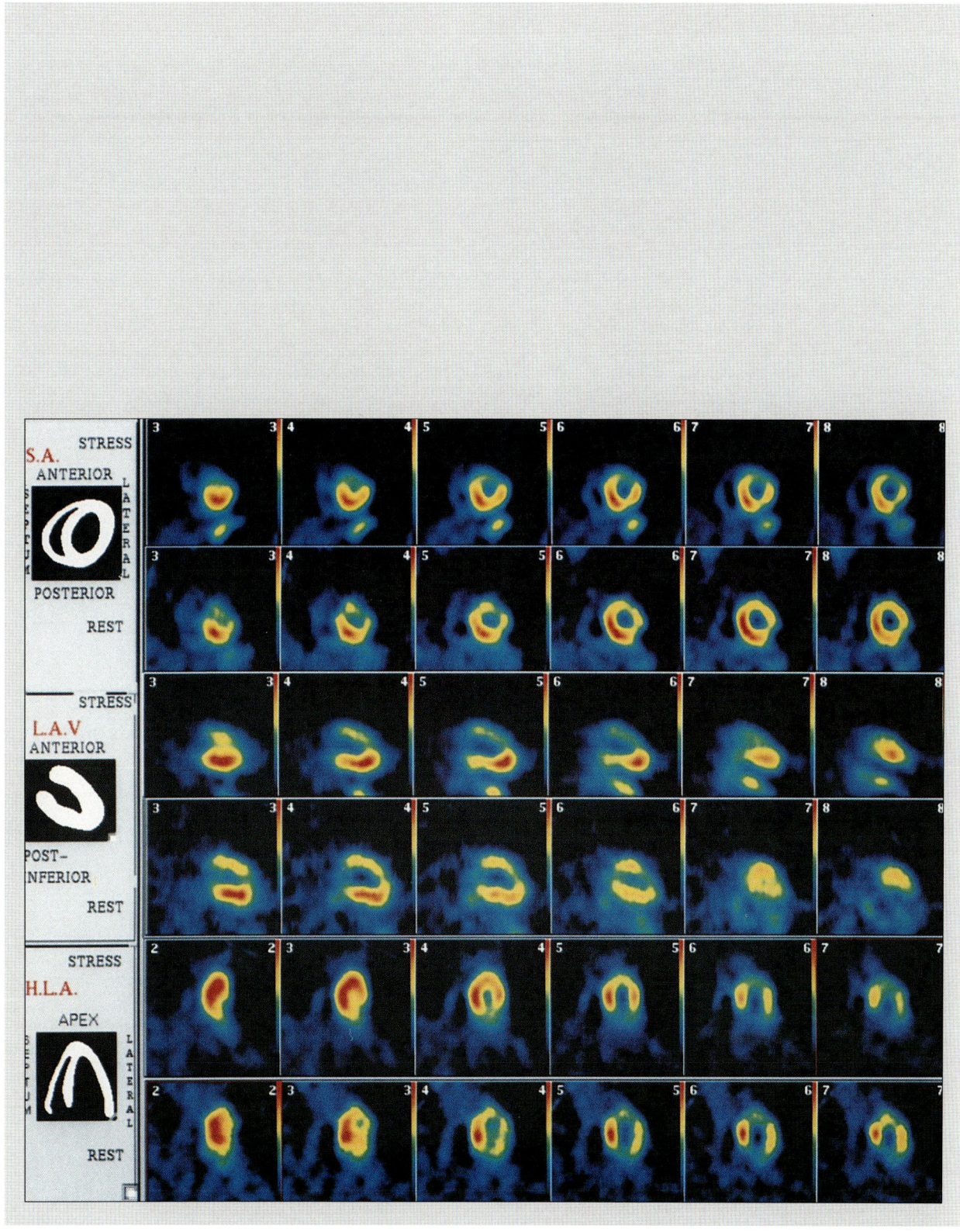

Figure 89 Same format in a patient with a previous anterior myocardial infarction. A perfusion defect is seen in the anterior wall of the short-axis views (top panel), which fills in or redistributes at rest (second panel down). A marked perfusion defect is seen in the anterior wall in the vertical long-axis views (third panel), which partially redistributes at rest (fourth panel). The patient was subsequently demonstrated to have two tight left anterior descending stenoses

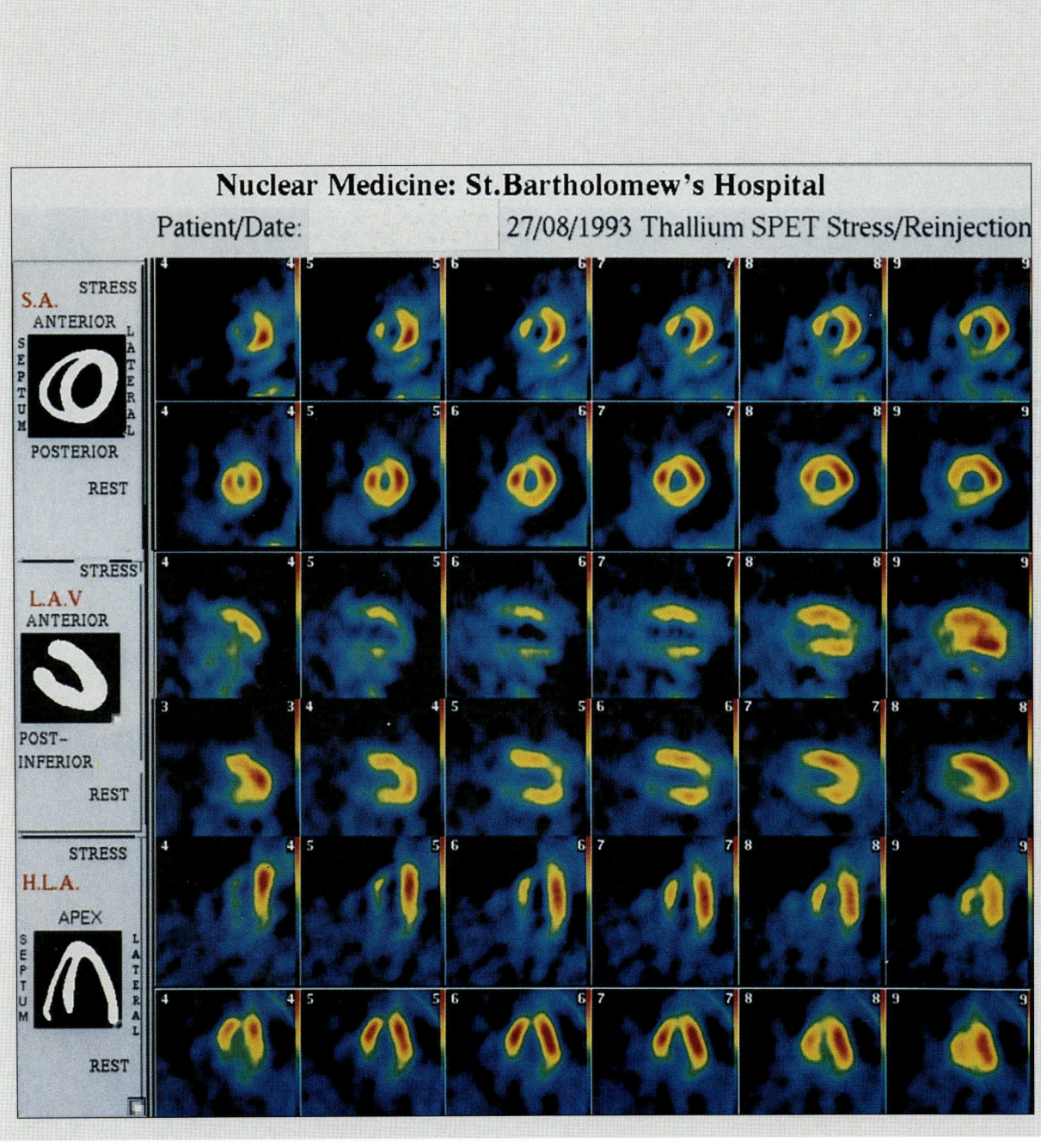

Figure 90 Same format in a patient with a previous apical infarction, best appreciated on the last horizontal panel but with severe inducible ischemia in the anteroseptal region (upper panel and fifth panel), and the anterior and inferior walls (third panel). The rest images in the second, fourth and sixth panels show only the small fixed defect at the apex. This profound inducible ischemia carries an adverse prognosis and the patient underwent surgical revascularization for triple vessel coronary disease

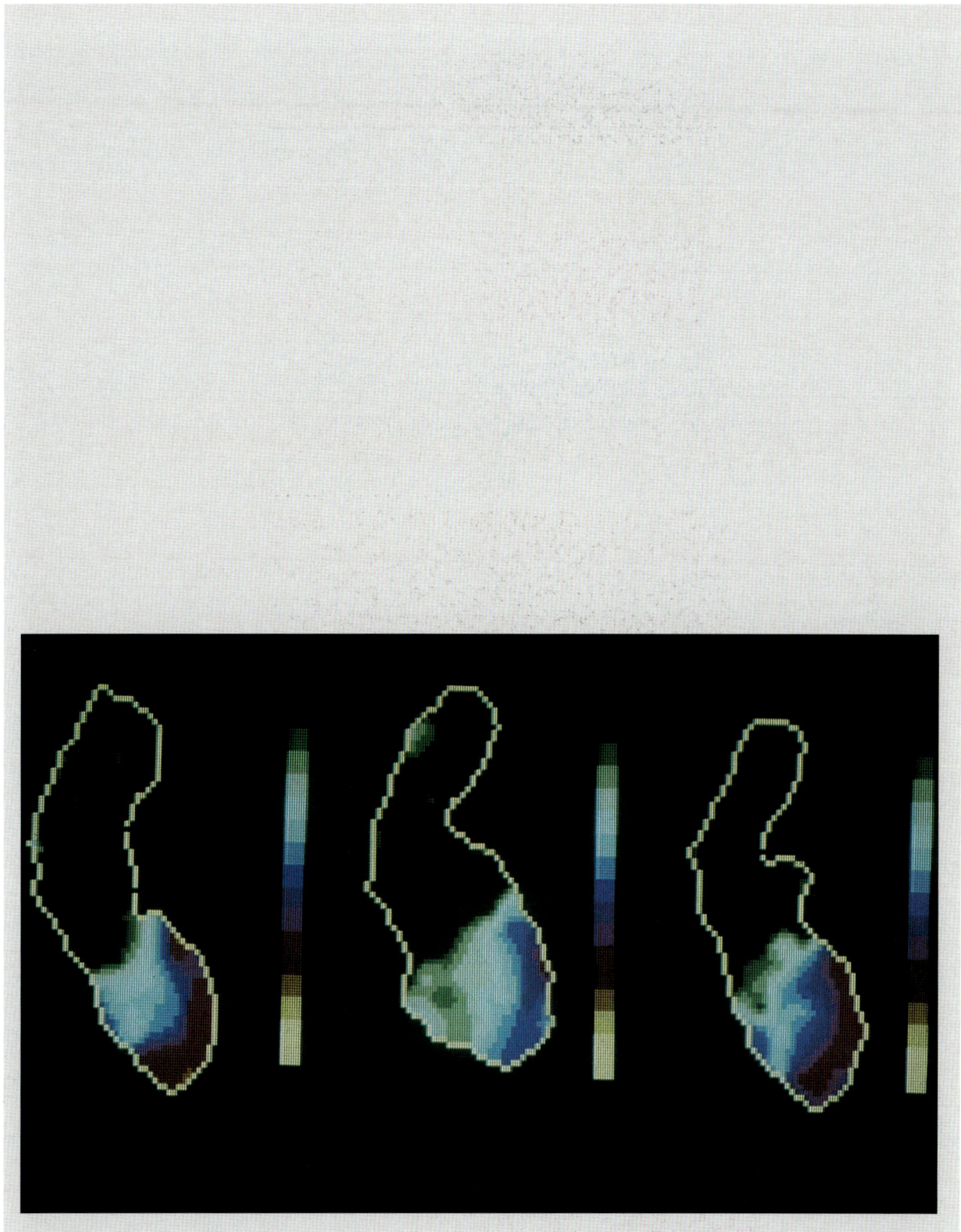

Figure 91 Regional ejection fraction images at rest (left hand), peak exercise (middle) and recovery (right hand) from a first-pass radionuclide angiogram. The format of the regional ejection fraction images is as described in Figures 81 and 82. Note the good function delineated by red in the anterior wall and apex in the outer two images, with the inferior wall shown in blue on these outer two images, indicating the previous infarction. On the middle image at peak exercise, the function in the anterior wall has also decreased, with blue replacing red. This patient had an occluded right coronary artery and a subtotal left anterior descending stenosis, the latter producing the regional wall abnormality at peak exercise. (Reprinted with permission from *American Journal of Cardiology*, 1984, **53**, 1532–7)

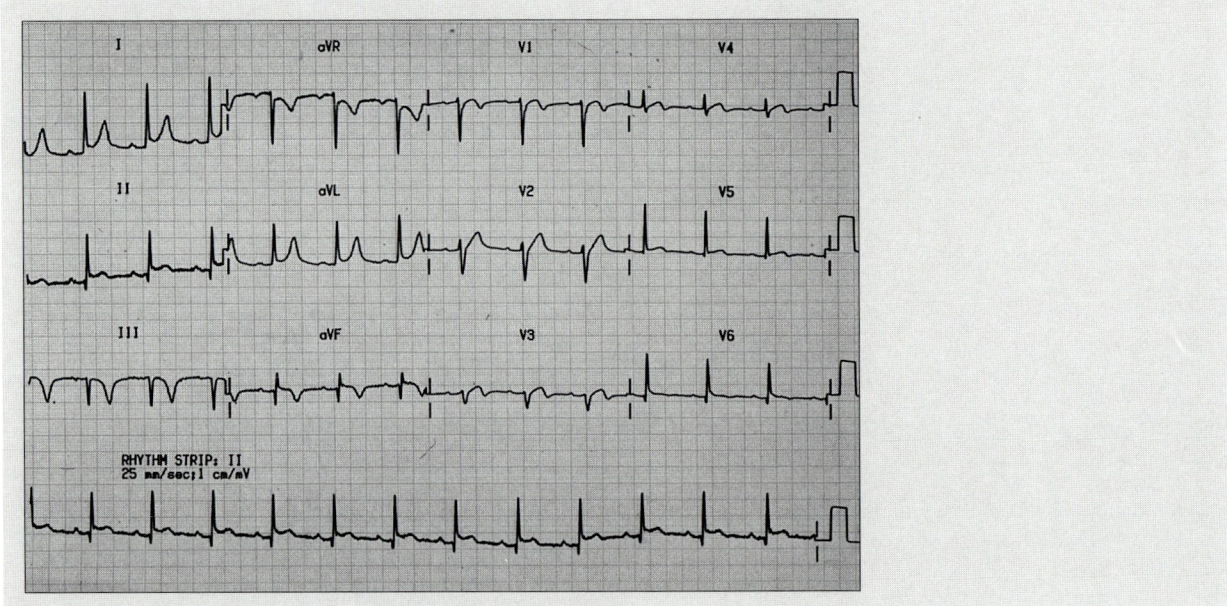

Figure 92 12-lead ECG in a patient convalescing from an acute myocardial infarction who developed more chest pain, worse with inspiration and postural change. There is concave ST segment elevation in leads I, AVL and V6 and some T wave changes anteriorly. The patient had a loud pericardial rub and these ECG changes represent pericarditis superimposed upon infarction

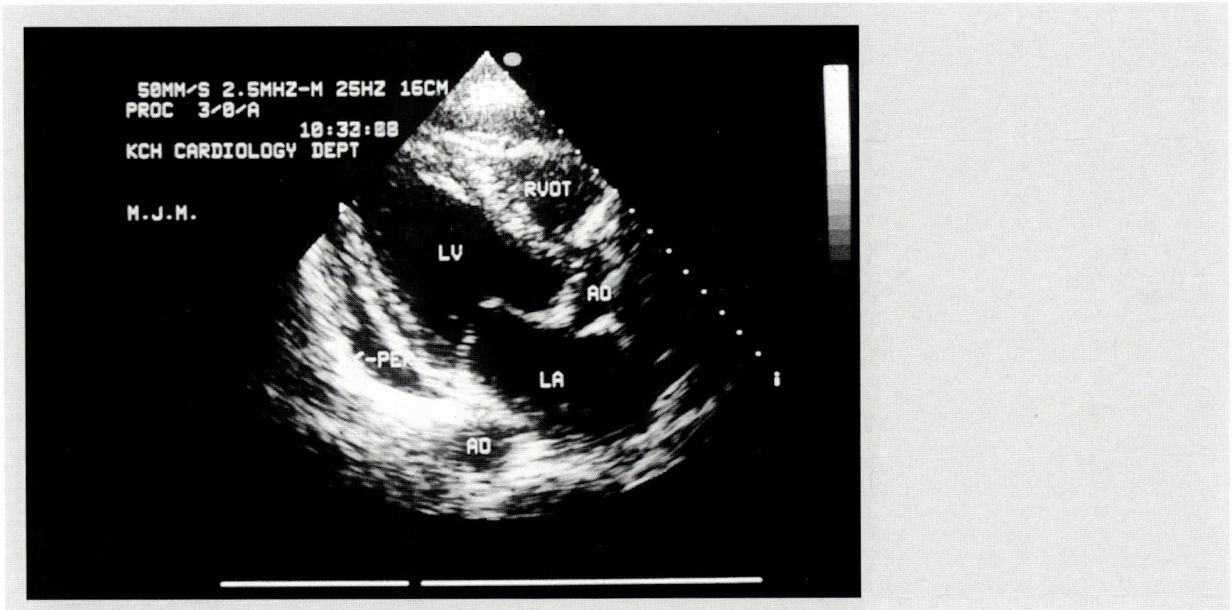

Figure 93 Two-dimensional echocardiogram in a long-axis view showing a pericardial effusion (PER) posterior to the left ventricle. Although pericarditis is often a transient phenomenon, prolonged pericardial effusions can occur and recur as part of Dressler's syndrome

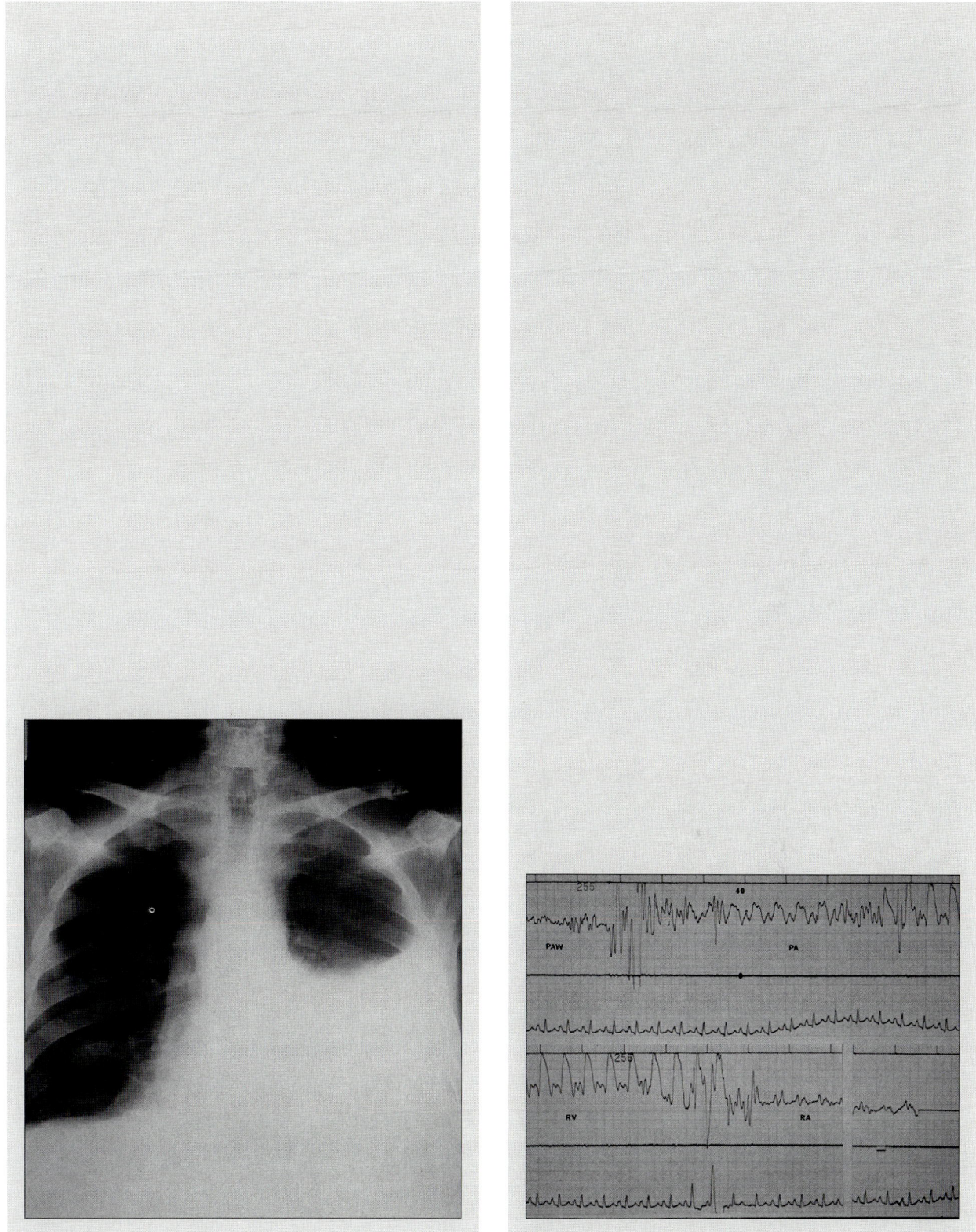

Figure 94 Chest X-ray from a patient with Dressler's syndrome. The patient had a pericardial effusion, a large left-sided pleural effusion, and a much smaller effusion (not well shown) on the right side

Figure 95 Pressure traces from the pulmonary capillary wedge through the pulmonary artery, right ventricle and right atrium showing the diastolic pressures equalizing in a case of constrictive pericarditis. This is an unusual complication of postinfarction pericardial effusion

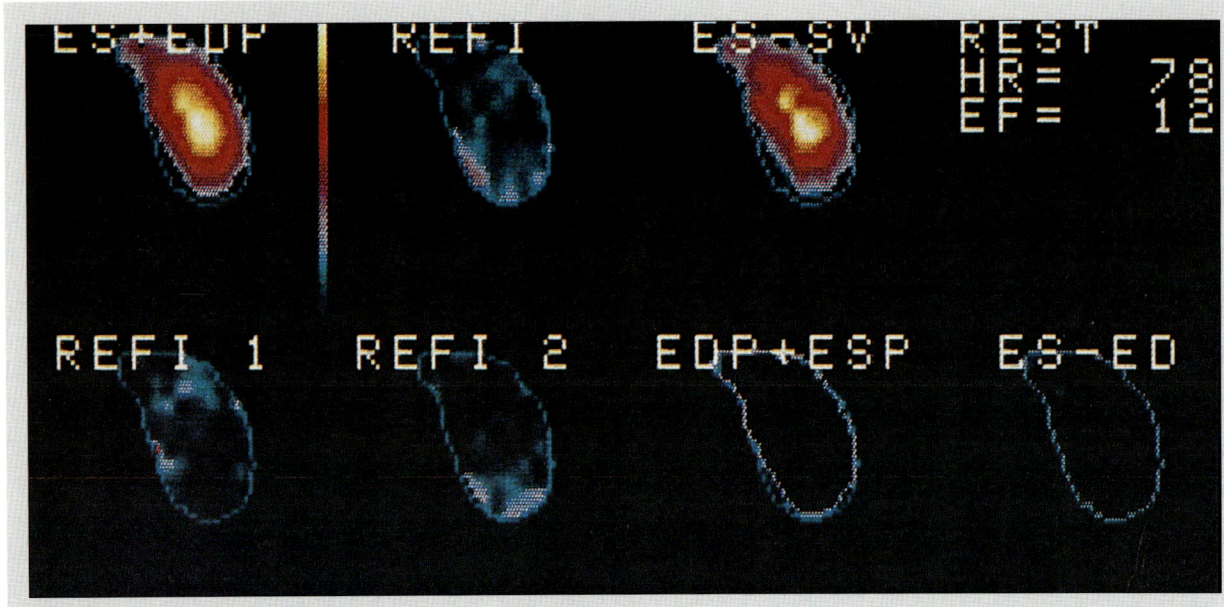

Figure 96 First-pass radionuclide scan in a patient with single vessel occlusion and extensive anterior infarction with expansion and an ejection fraction of only 12%. Note there is hardly any wall motion and global dysfunction. This patient was in cardiogenic shock with a systolic blood pressure of 80 mmHg, sweating, confusion and oliguria

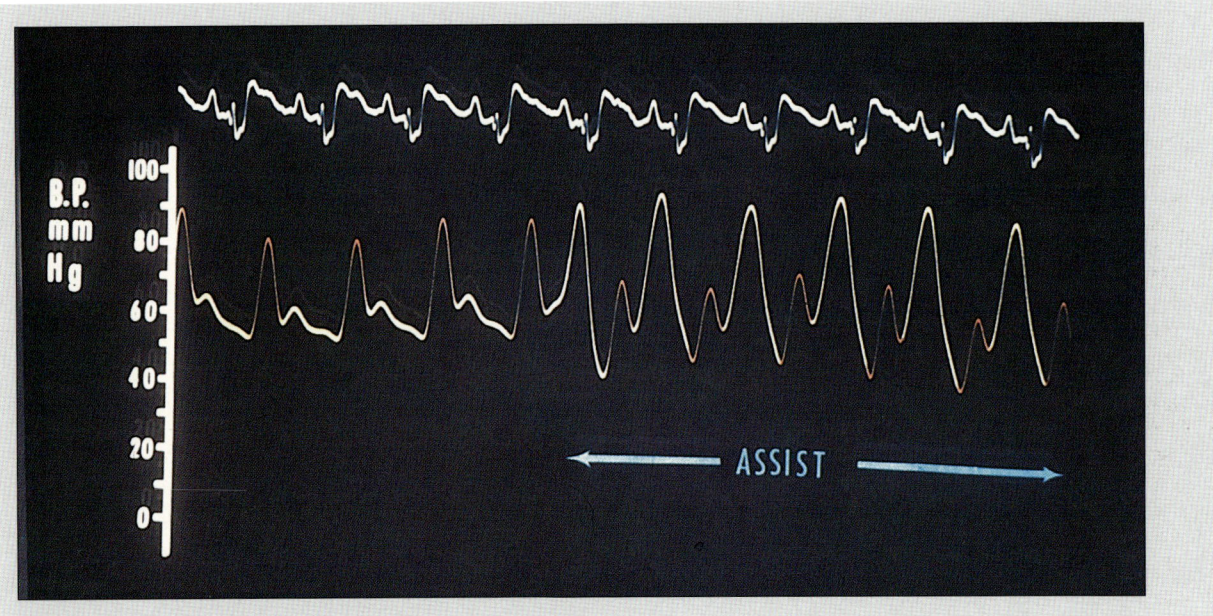

Figure 97 Arterial pressure trace showing low systolic blood pressure (first four beats), but when intraortic balloon pumping is instituted there is augmentation of the diastolic pressure to 90 mmHg and over). Note also the dip after each diastolic augmentation which leads to a reduction in afterload

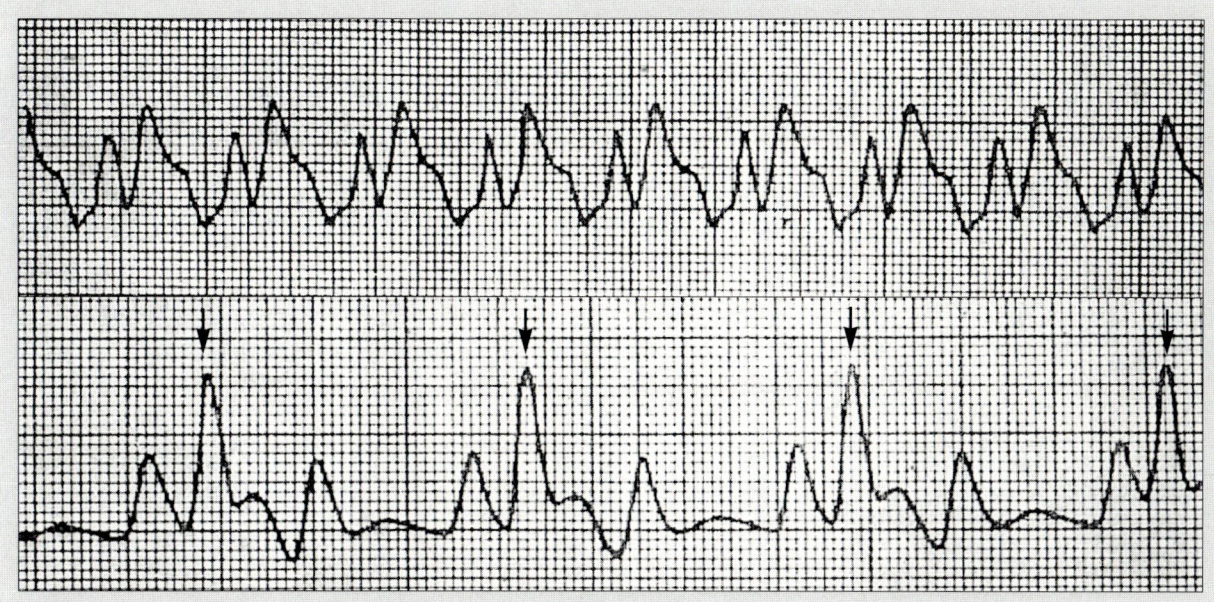

Figure 98 Another example of balloon pump augmentation of diastolic pressure and afterload reduction. The top panel shows the balloon pump working on a one-to-one basis. The lower panel shows the balloon pump working on every alternate beat (arrowed)

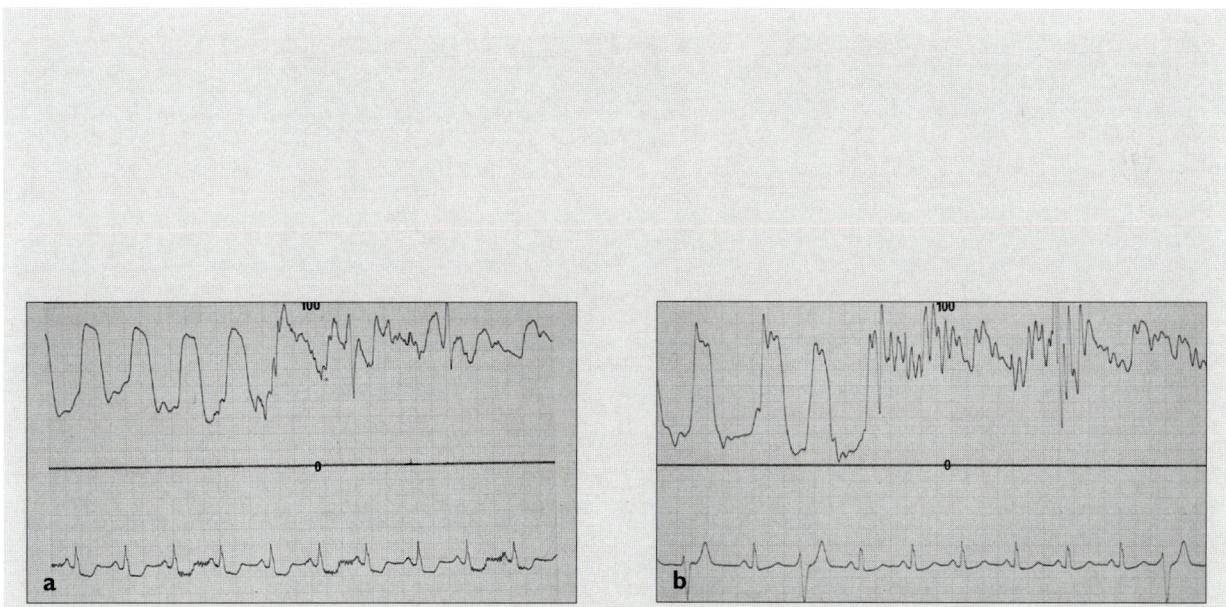

Figure 99 Left ventricular and aortic pressure traces (a) pre and (b) post intraortic balloon pump assist. Note the left ventricular and diastolic pressure is up to 40 mmHg, before the balloon pump is working, and down to between 8 and 12 mmHg when the balloon pump is assisting

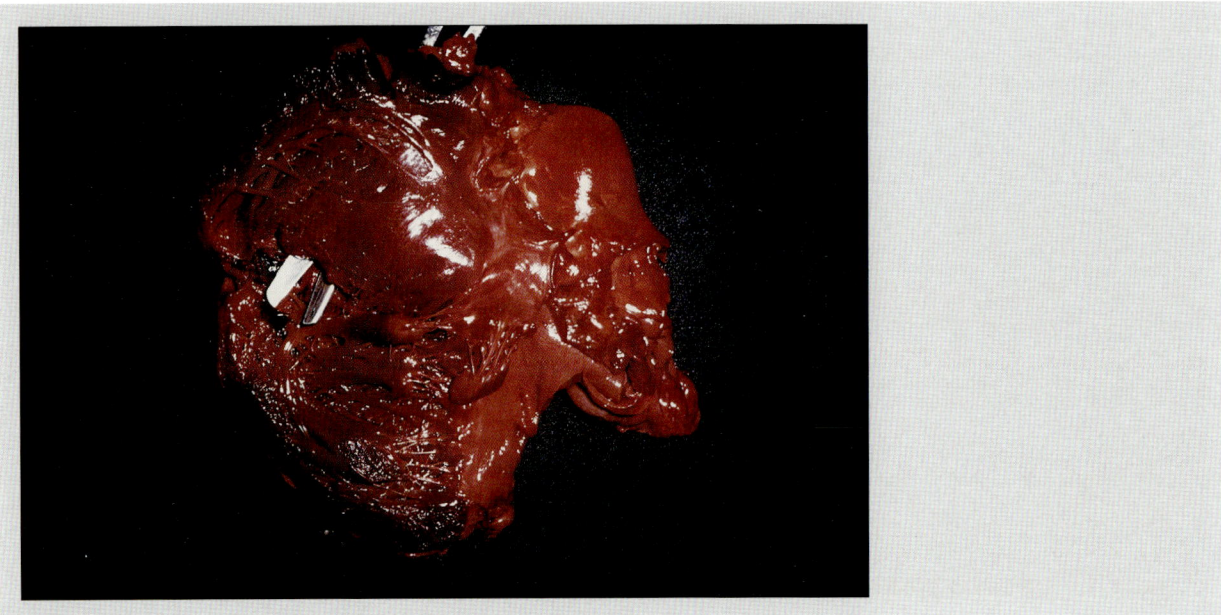

Figure 100 Postmortem heart with a pair of forceps passed through a tear in the interventricular septum, i.e. a postinfarct ventricular septal defect

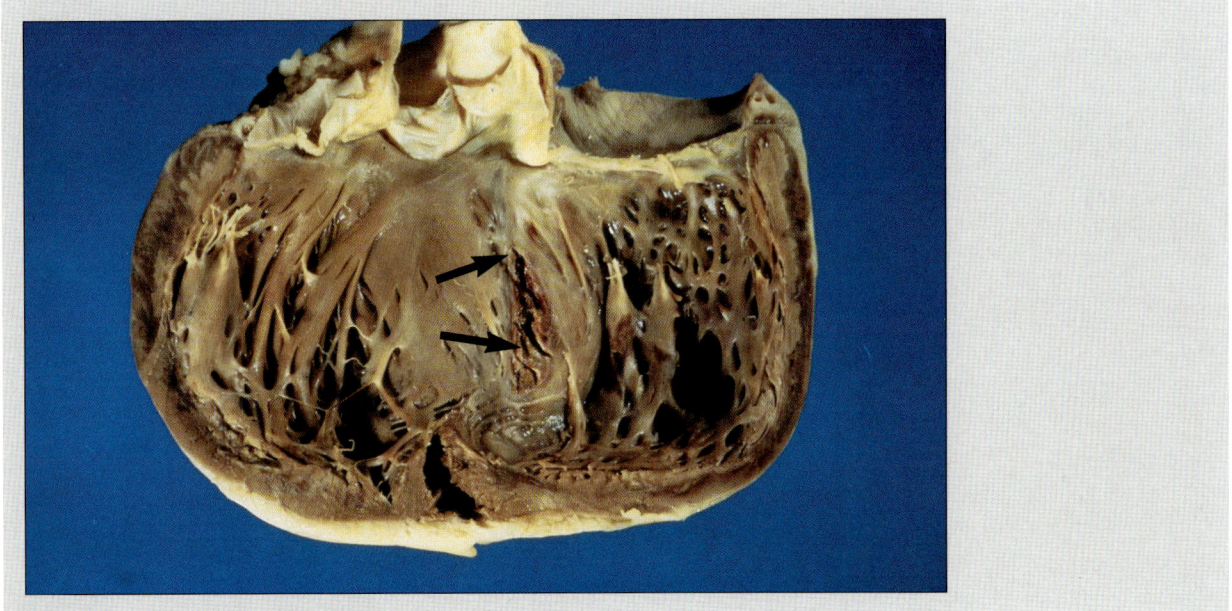

Figure 101 Another example of a postmortem heart showing a longitudinal tear in the septum (arrowed) and a postinfarct ventricular septal defect

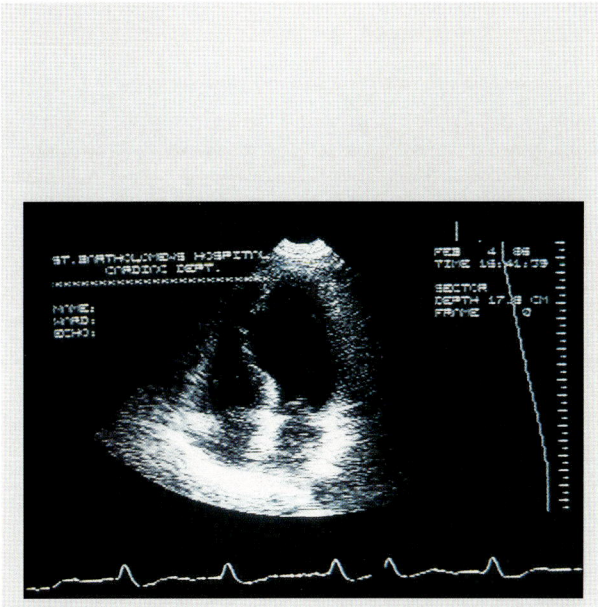

Figure 102 Two-dimensional echocardiogram in the apical four-chamber view showing a defect in the intraventricular septum postinfarction

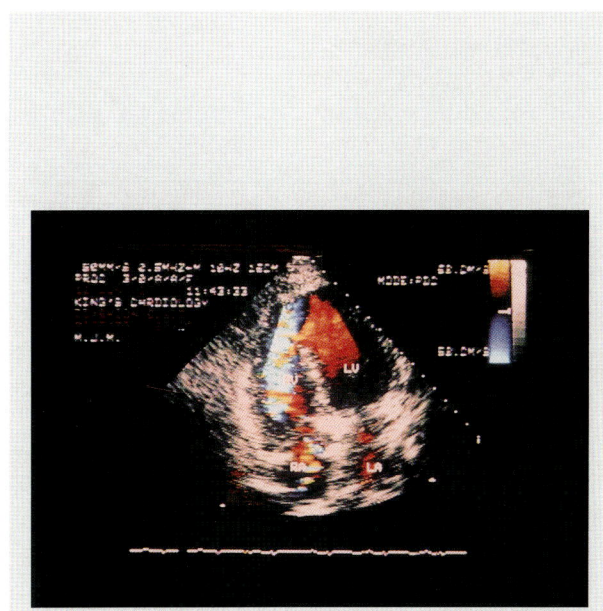

Figure 103 Two-dimensional echocardiogram and color flow Doppler study of a postinfarct ventricular septal defect. The signal colored red from the left ventricle is seen passing across the defect in the septum; the signal from the right ventricle is colored blue

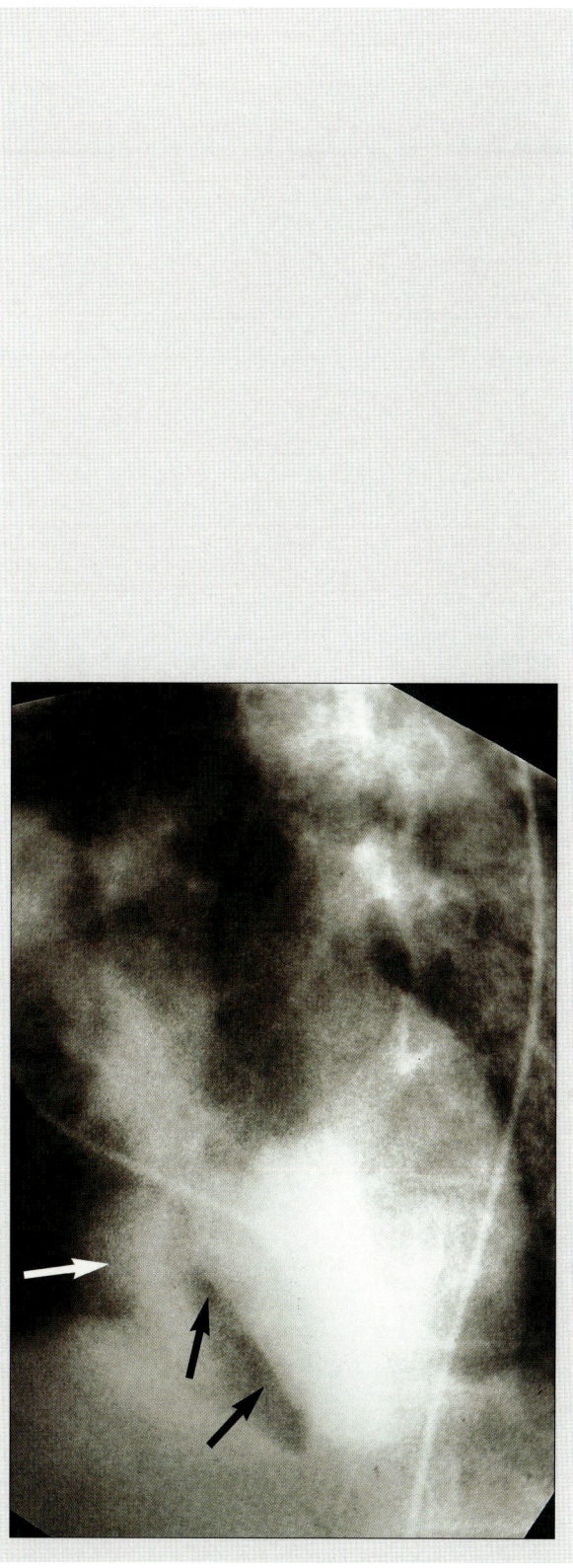

Figure 104 Contrast angiogram from a patient with a postinfarction ventricular septum defect. The catheter is in the left ventricle in the left anterior oblique projection with cranial angulation. To the left of the left ventricle is the interventricular septum shown as a radiolucent area (black arrows), and contrast in the right ventricle is shown to the left of the septum (white arrow)

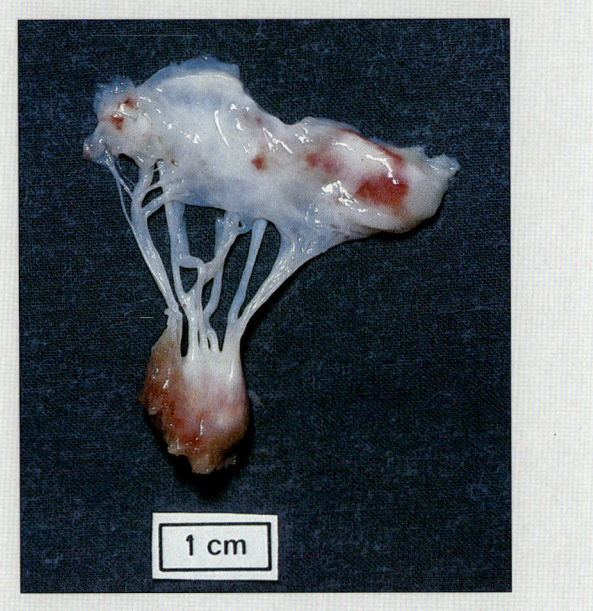

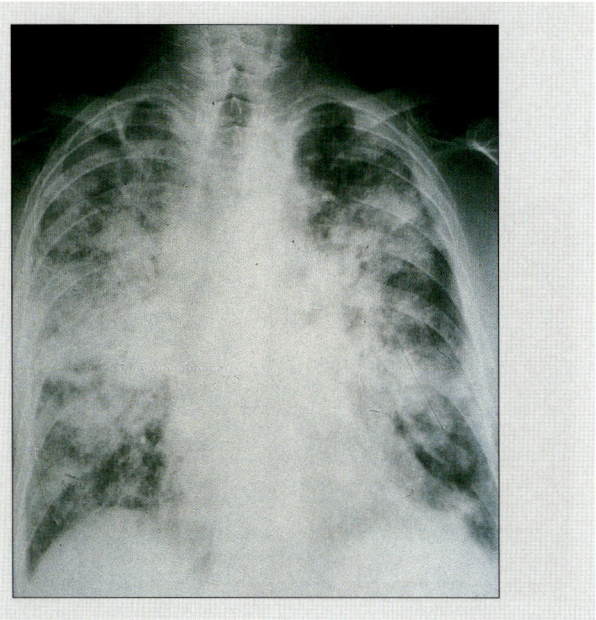

Figure 105 Postmortem specimen of infarcted ruptured papillary muscle leading to overwhelming mitral regurgitation and sudden death. The chordae tendineae are seen above the ruptured papillary muscle; hemorrhagic infarction of the papillary muscle itself is clearly seen

Figure 106 Posteroanterior chest X-ray in a patient with acute ischemic mitral regurgitation showing overwhelming pulmonary edema

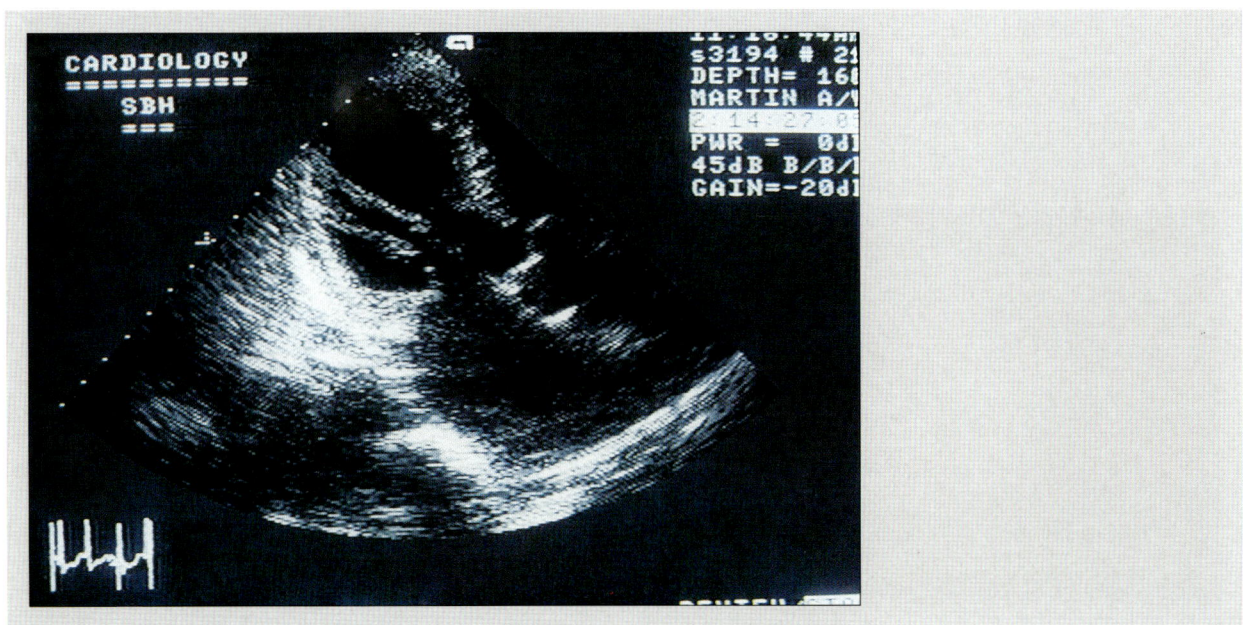

Figure 107 Two-dimensional echocardiogram showing ruptured papillary muscle waving freely in the left ventricle

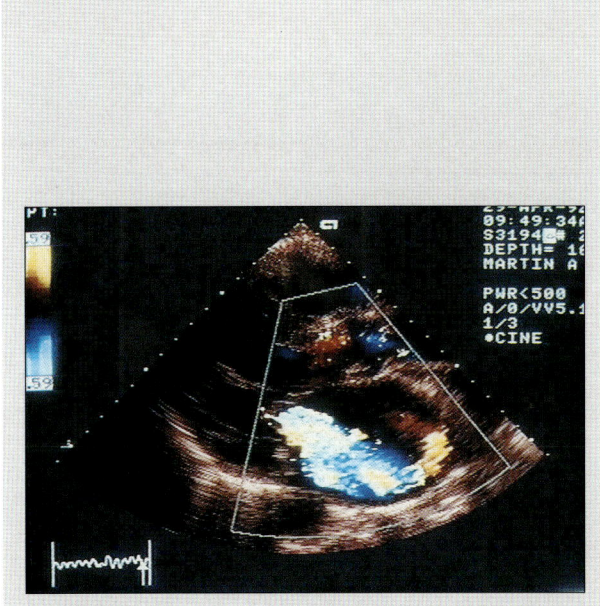

Figure 108 Long-axis two-dimensional echocardiogram with color flow Doppler showing large yellow flame of mitral regurgitation filling the left atrium in systole

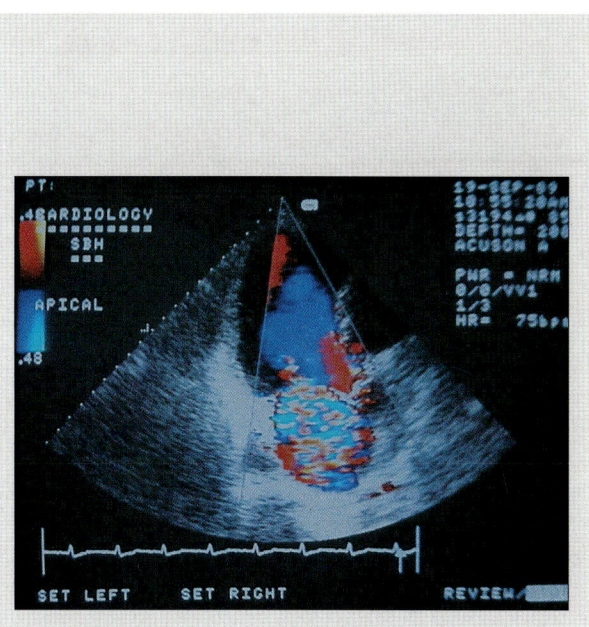

Figure 109 Apical two-chamber view of severe mitral regurgitation after an infarction. The left atrium is full of multicolored signal indicating aliaising and turbulent flow

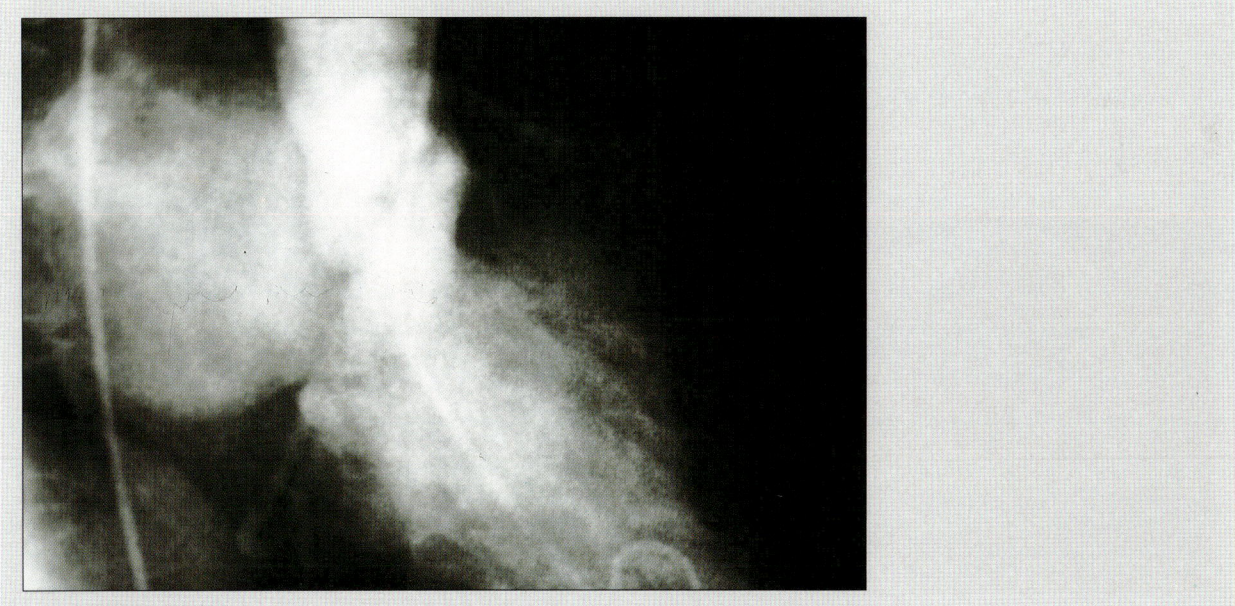

Figure 110 Contrast angiogram of left ventricle showing severe mitral regurgitation into the left atrium. In this situation the left atrium is often small and non-compliant and unable to absorb small changes in volume without a rise in pressure

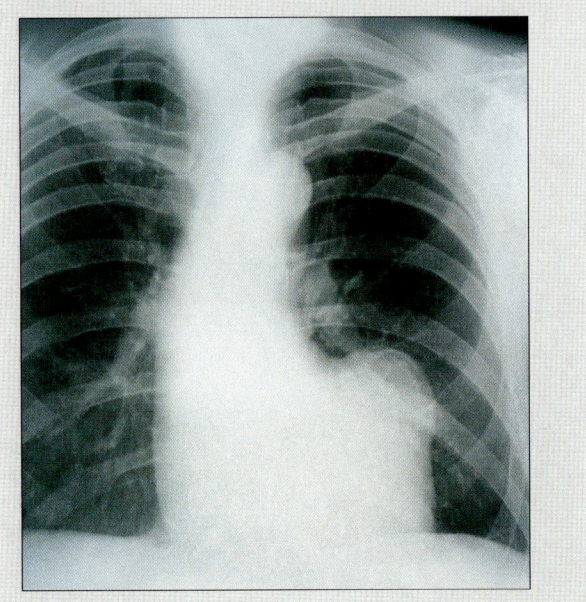

Figure 111 Posteroanterior chest X-ray showing large abnormal bulge on left heart border, indicating left ventricular aneurysm. Note that at least 50% of aneurysms do not produce this abnormality on chest X-ray

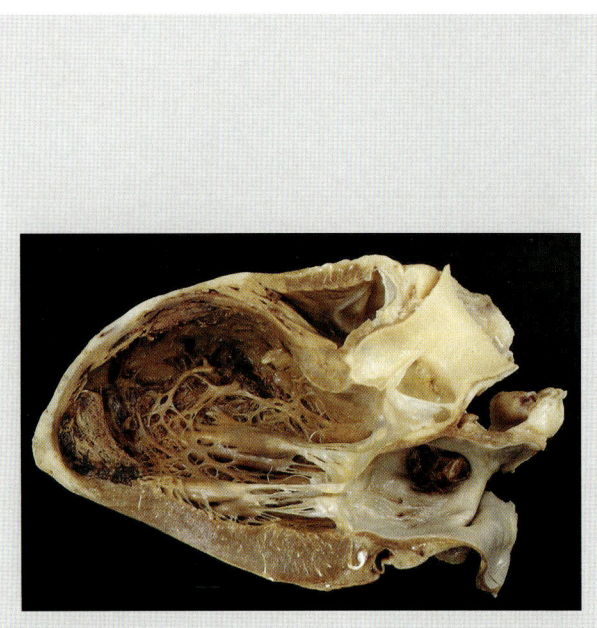

Figure 112 Postmortem section showing a long-axis cut of an expanding thinned anterior myocardial infarction with thrombus at the apex. There is also some thrombus in the left atrium. It is thought that this infarct expansion and thinning may produce left ventricular aneurysms. Note that the posterior wall is normal. The attachments of the mitral valve are clearly seen

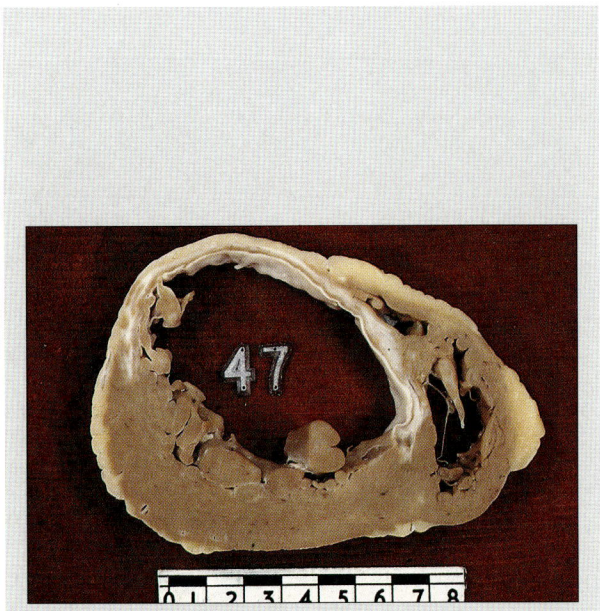

Figure 113 Cross-section of a postmortem heart showing old anterior and septal infarction consisting of white fibrous tissue with thinning and expansion of the infarcted territory

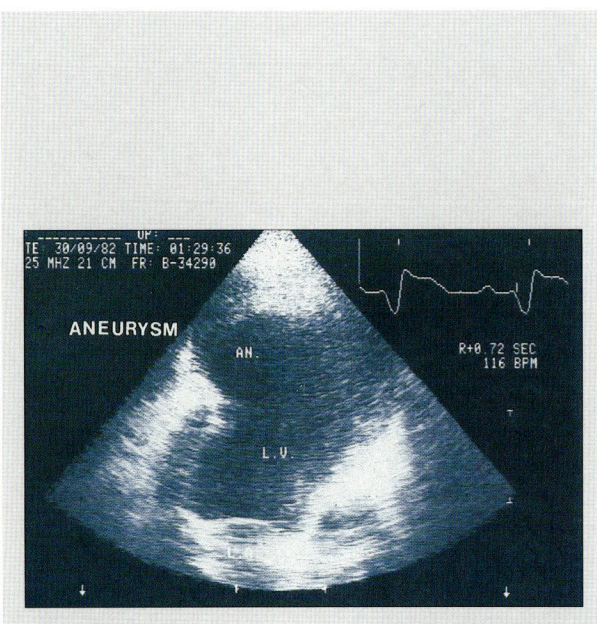

Figure 114 Two-dimensional echocardiogram showing the left ventricular cavity with a large apical aneurysm (AN)

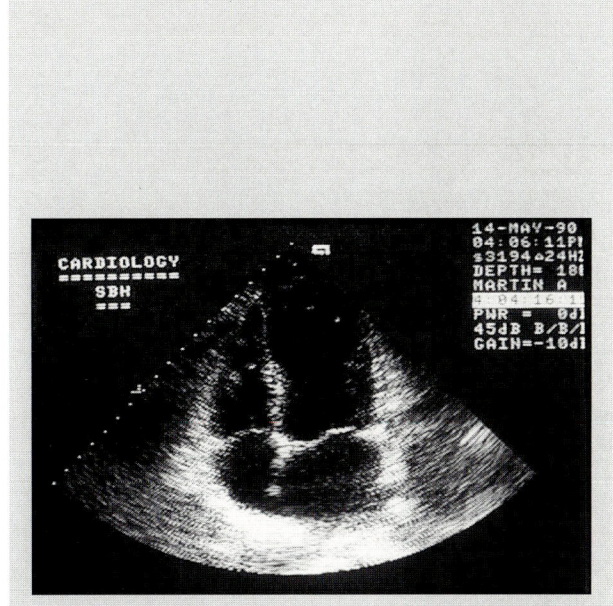

Figure 115 Apical four-chamber view showing a left ventricular aneurysm at the apex. Note how the upper part of the interventricular septum and posterior wall thicken normally and how thin are the echoes from the aneurysmal segment towards the apex

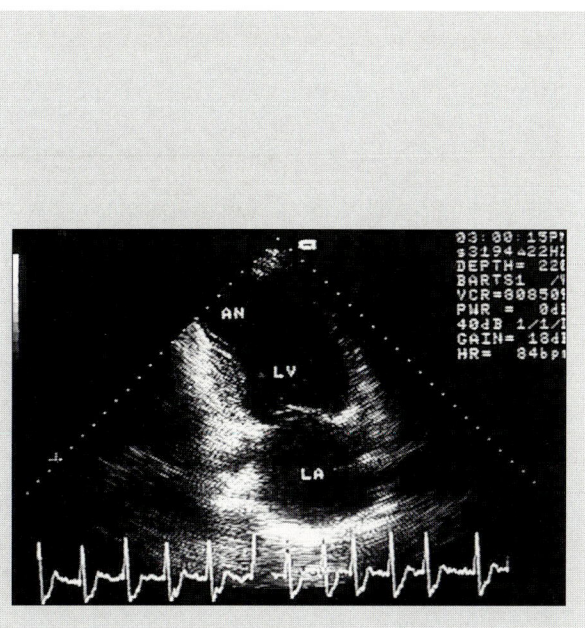

Figure 116 Another example of a large apical left ventricular aneurysm on the apical two-chamber view of two-dimensional echo

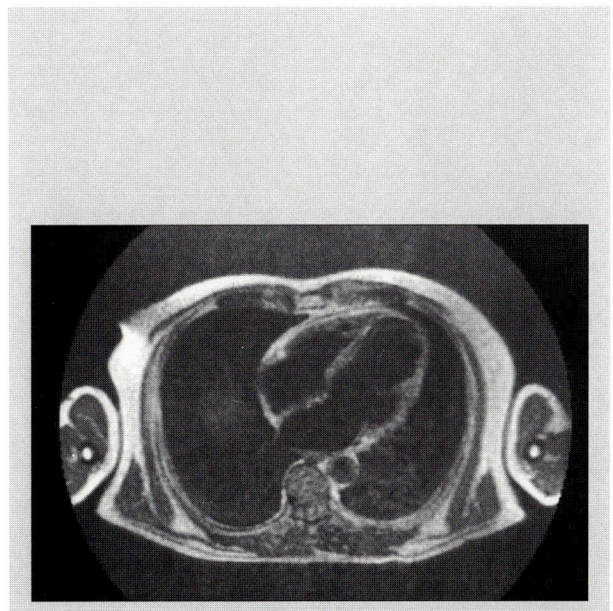

Figure 117 Magnetic resonance transverse spin echo image at end-diastole in a patient with a previous anterior infarction and left anterior descending occlusion. This image shows thinning of the apical myocardium with normal thickness of the basal parts of the septum and lateral wall

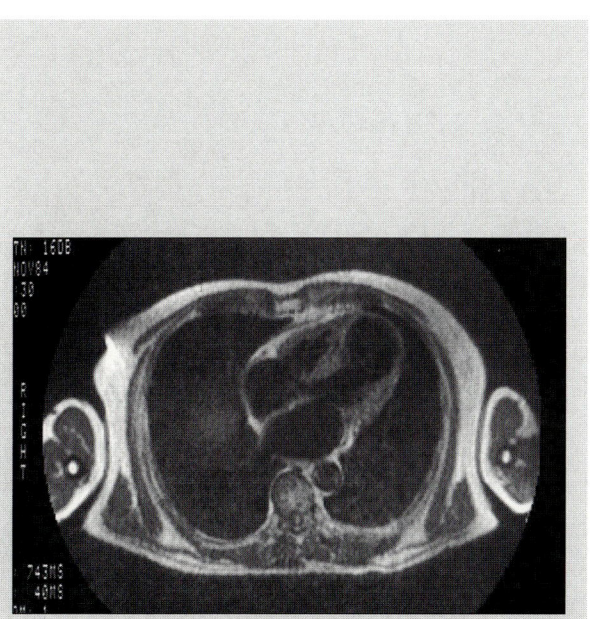

Figure 118 End-systolic image from the same patient as in Figure 117 showing normal thickening and contraction of the basal myocardium but paradoxical motion at the apex

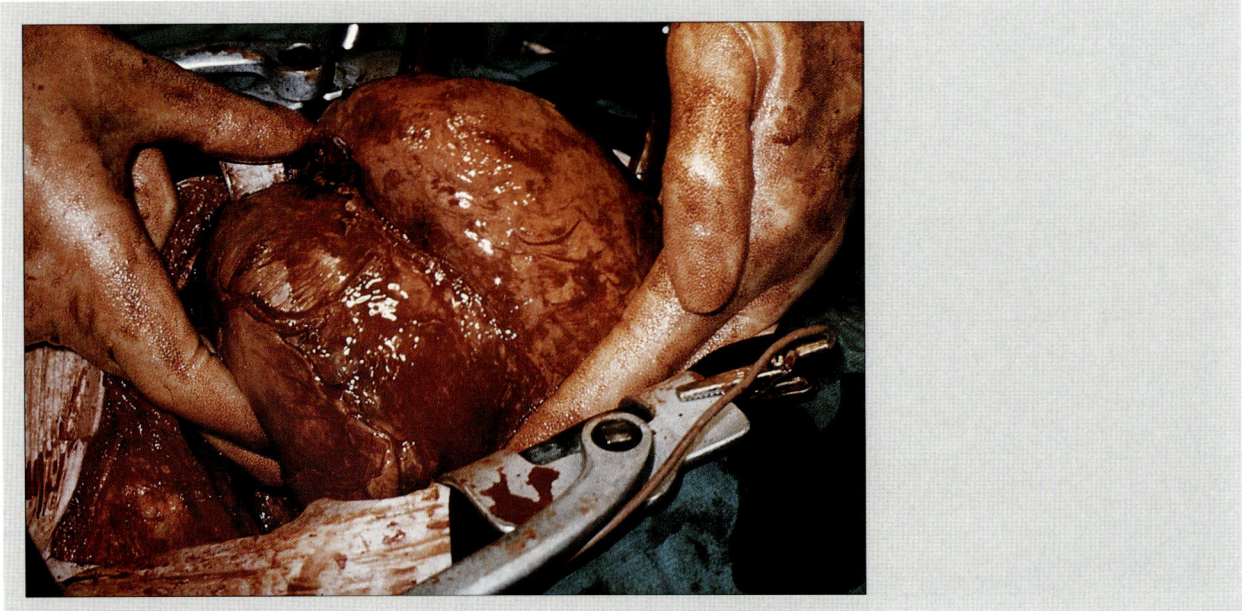

Figure 119 Large left ventricular aneurysm at operation

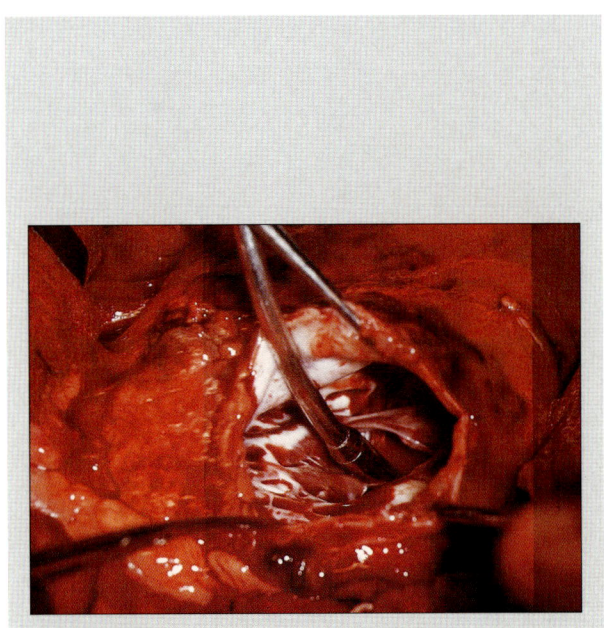

Figure 120 Aneurysm resection. Note the white endocardial fibrous tissue inside the aneurysm

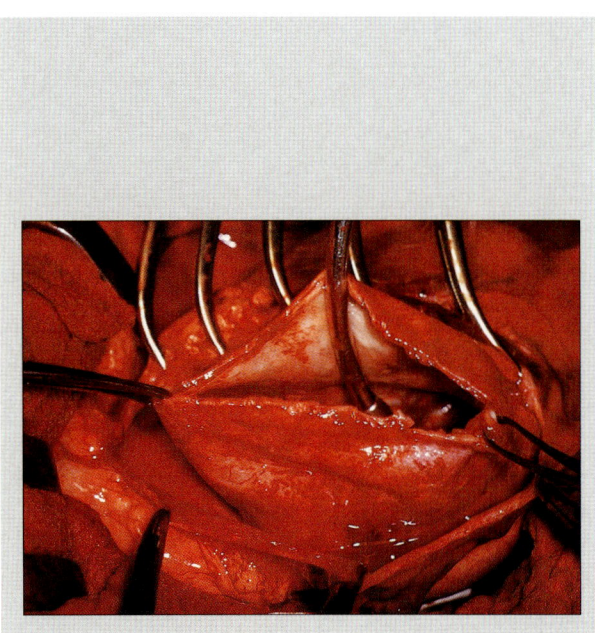

Figure 121 Margins of the aneurysm prior to closure of the aneurysmectomy site

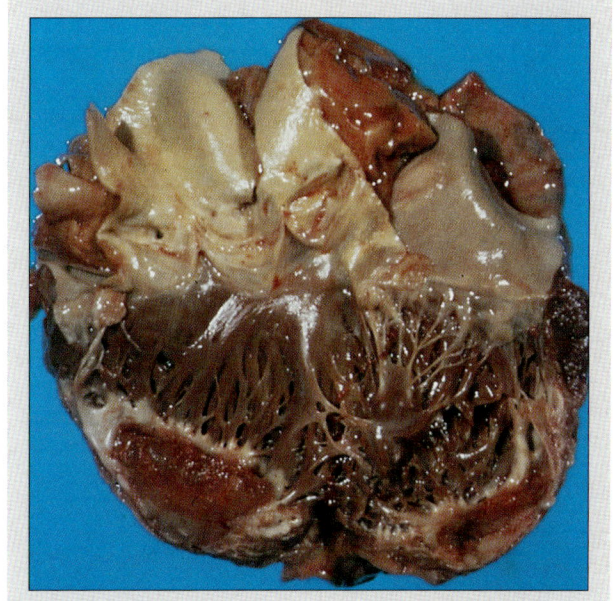

Figure 122 Postmortem heart showing a large apical aneurysm with white endocardial scarring in which is contained fresh thrombus

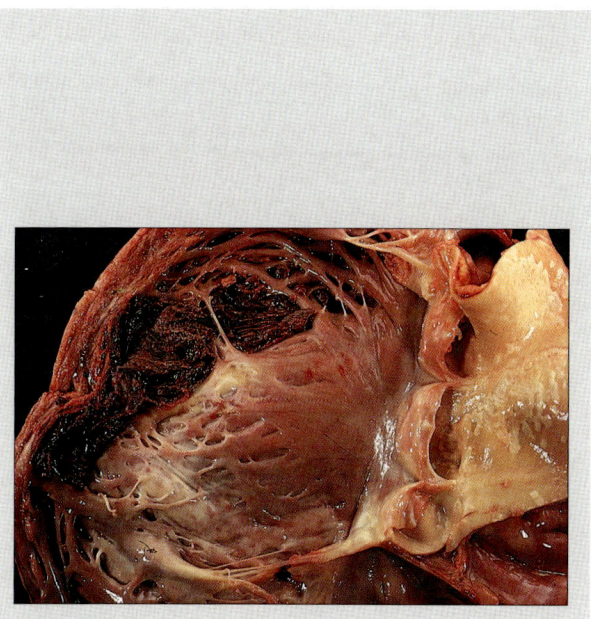

Figure 123 Long-axis cut of postmortem heart showing much adherent fresh thrombus

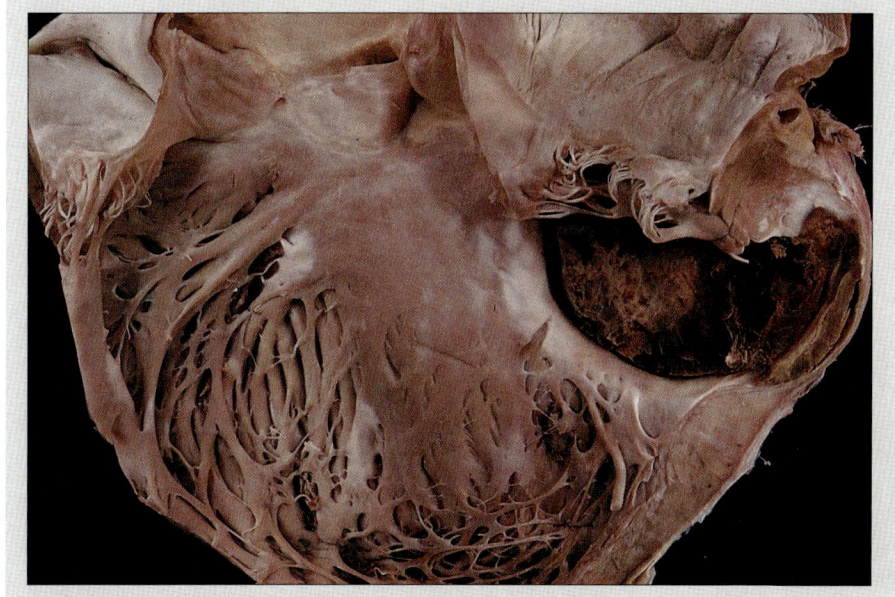

Figure 124 Posterior infarction with some old mural thrombus posteriorly

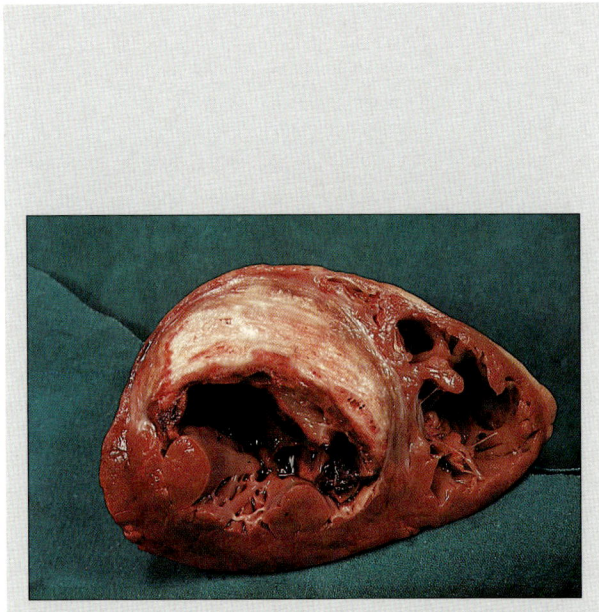

Figure 125 Postmortem heart showing a large mural thrombus which is white and rich in fibrin and platelets but poor in red blood cells in a recent 'expanding' infarction with thinning of the myocardium anteriorly

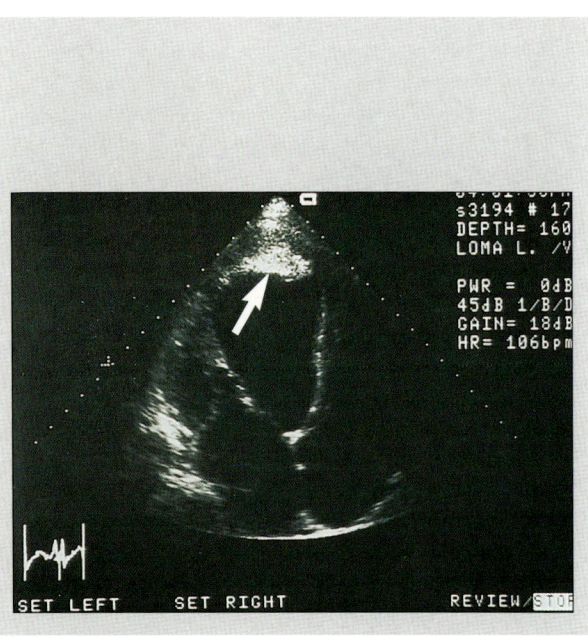

Figure 126 Two-dimensional echocardiogram showing dense echogenic mass of mural thrombus at the apex of the left ventricle (arrowed)

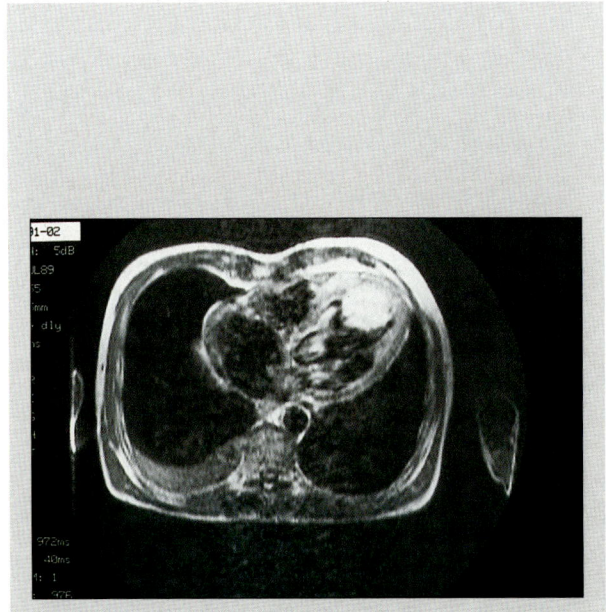

Figure 127 Spin echo magnetic resonance image from a patient with a previous anterior infarction and apical thrombus. The spin echo image shows the fresh thrombus as a very high signal at the apex. There is a signal from slowly moving blood towards the base of the ventricle

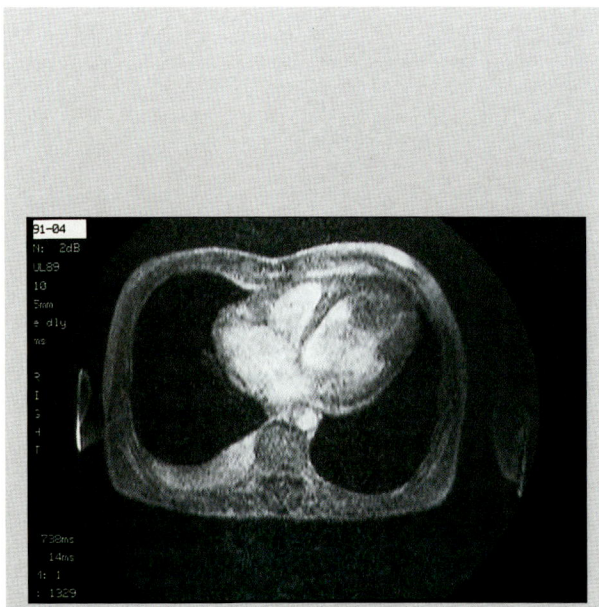

Figure 128 Gradient echo transverse image in the same patient as in Figure 127. Gradient image shows the thrombus as a relatively low signal compared with the higher signal from blood

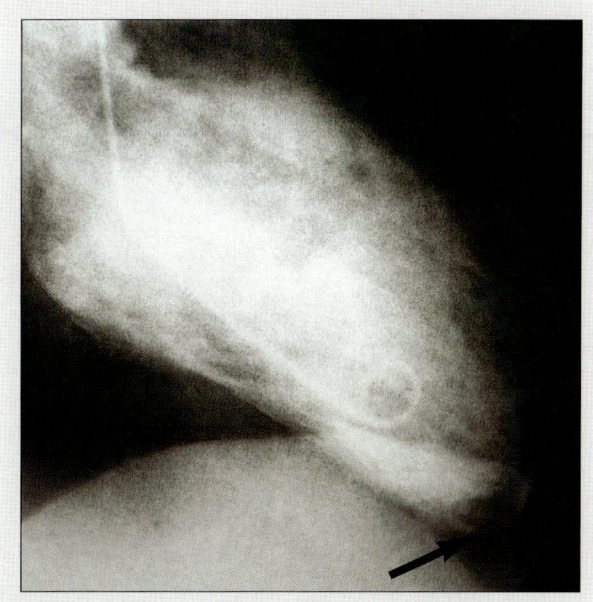

Figure 129 Frame from a left ventricular contrast angiogram in a patient 3 days after a sizeable anterior myocardial infarction. The filling defect at the apex of the left ventricle beyond the tip of the catheter represents fresh mural thrombus (arrowed)

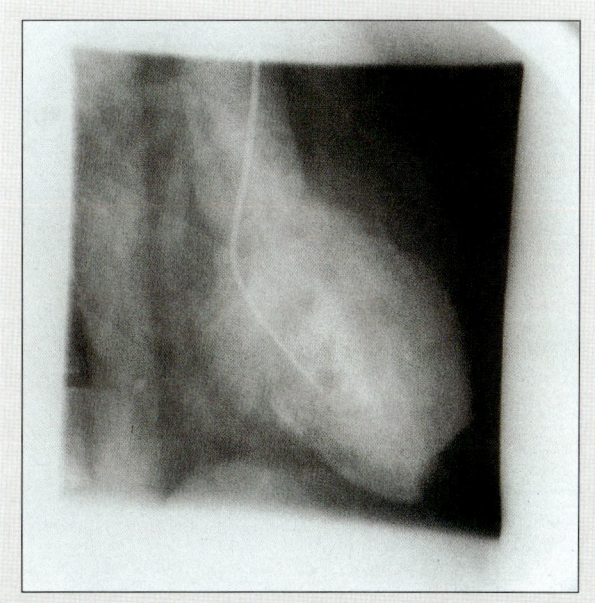

Figure 130 Frame from contrast angiogram in a patient with an anterior myocardial infarction 3 years previously. The filling defect at the apex represents old laminated thrombus

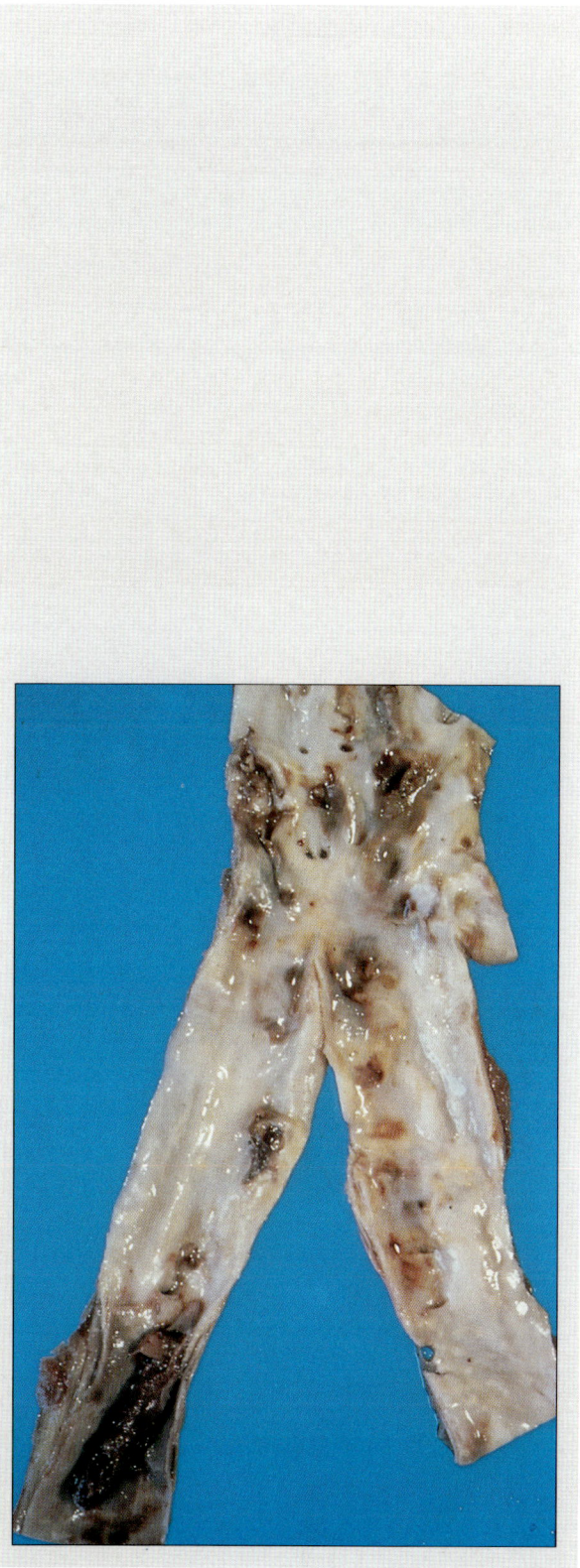

Figure 131 Postmortem specimen showing large embolus from mural thrombus to the right common iliac artery

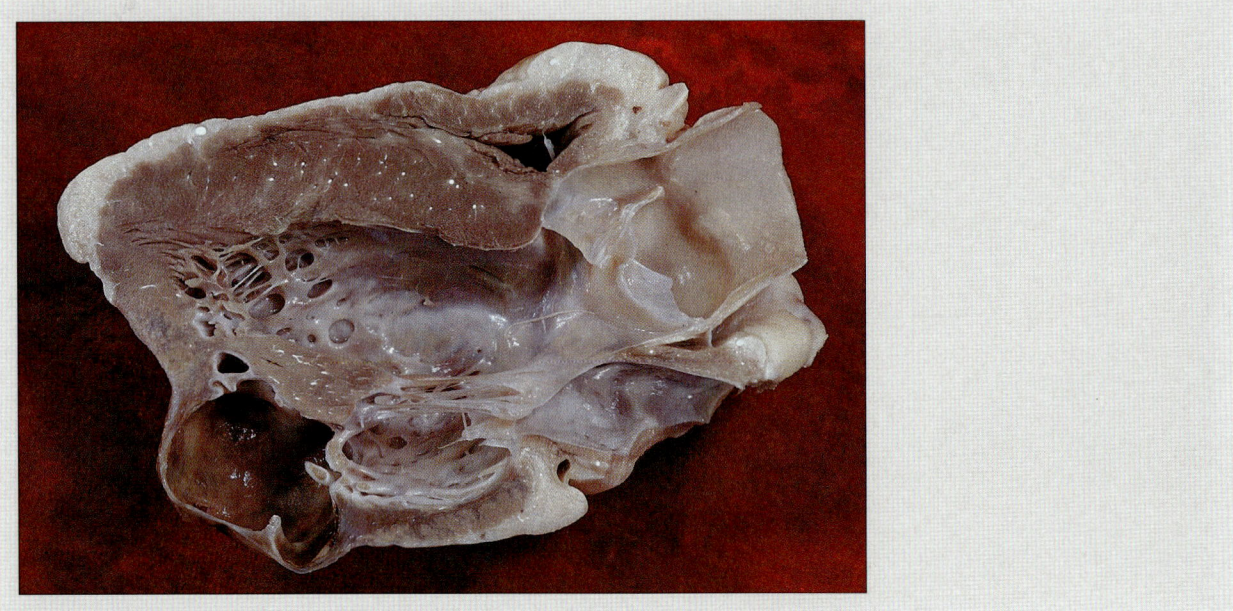

Figure 132 Long-axis cut through a posterior wall aneurysm which is very well localized and does not involve the entire posterior wall

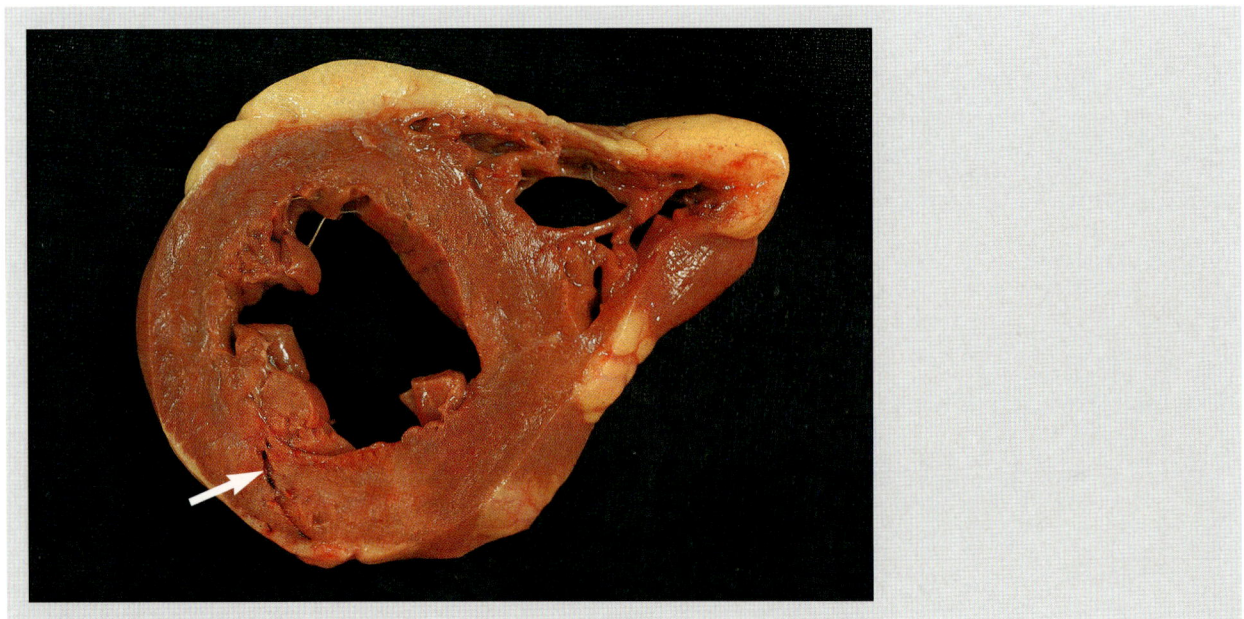

Figure 133 Postmortem heart from a recent posterior infarction with a longitudinal rupture clearly seen (arrowed)

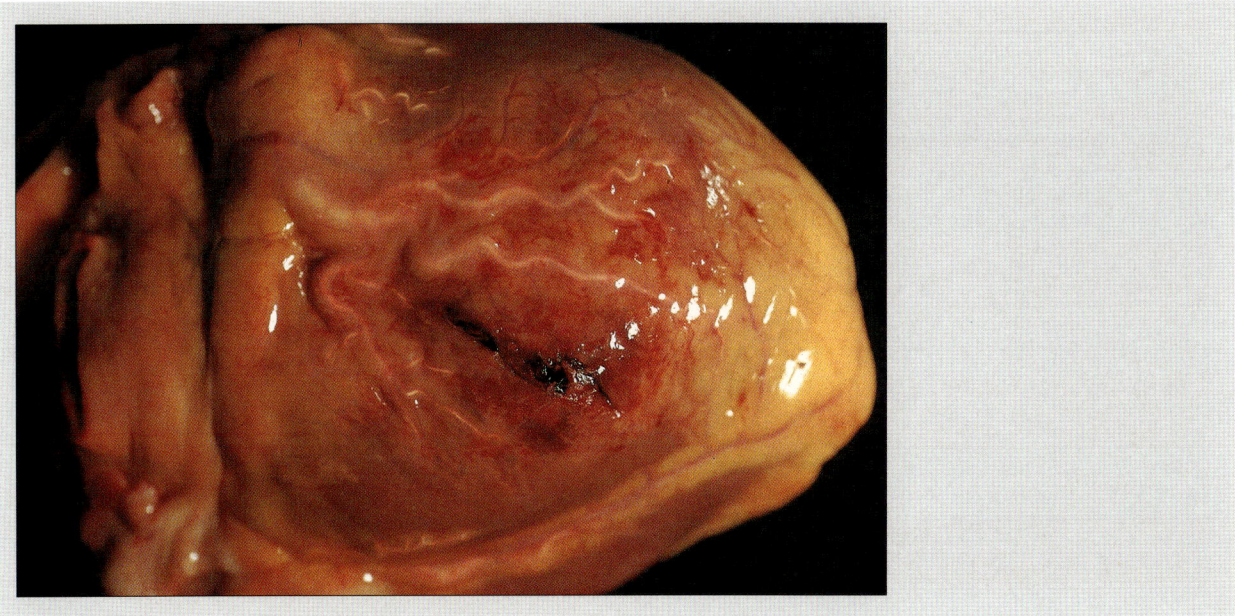

Figure 134 Extensive rupture of the posterior wall. Hemorrhage is seen on the surface of the heart

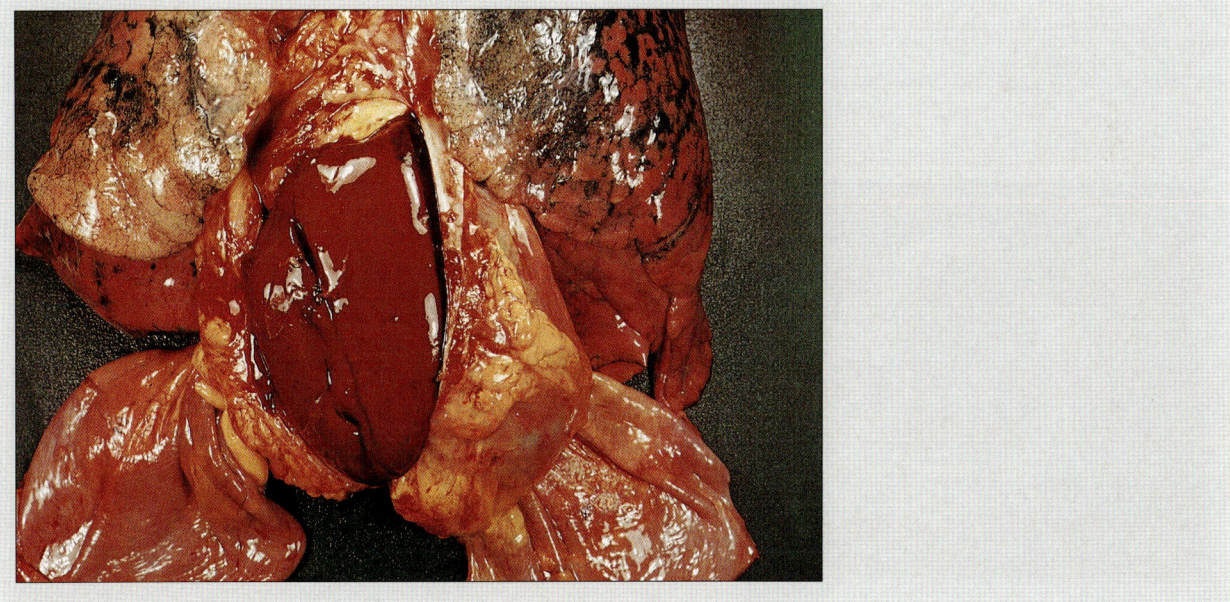

Figure 135 Massive hemopericardium secondary to myocardial rupture

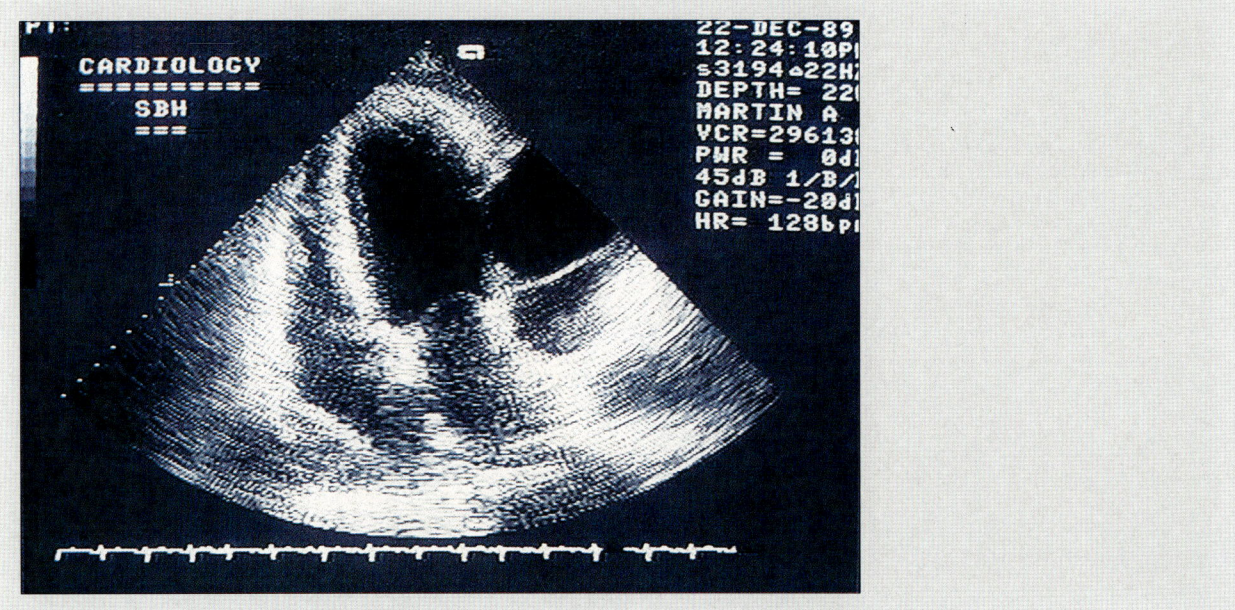

Figure 136 Two-dimensional echocardiogram showing an apical four-chamber view and a clear rupture of the free wall

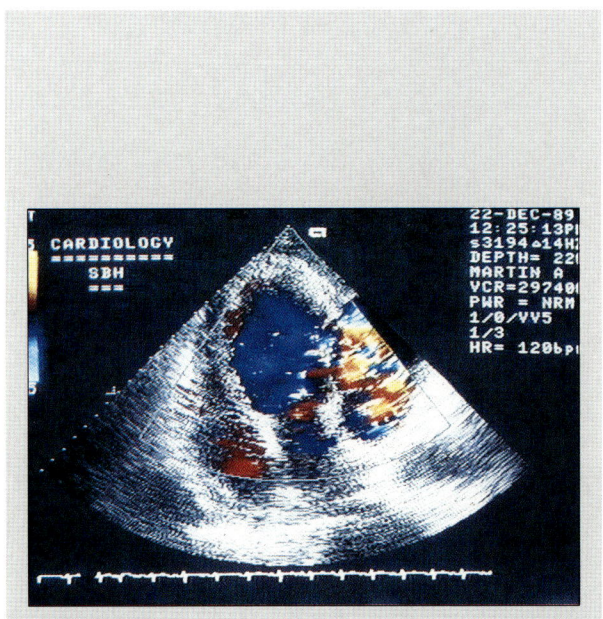

Figure 137 Color flow Doppler study at end-systole in the same patient as in Figure 136. The signal is seen streaming through the free wall rupture with a bright yellow signal in the pericardial sac which contains the rupture

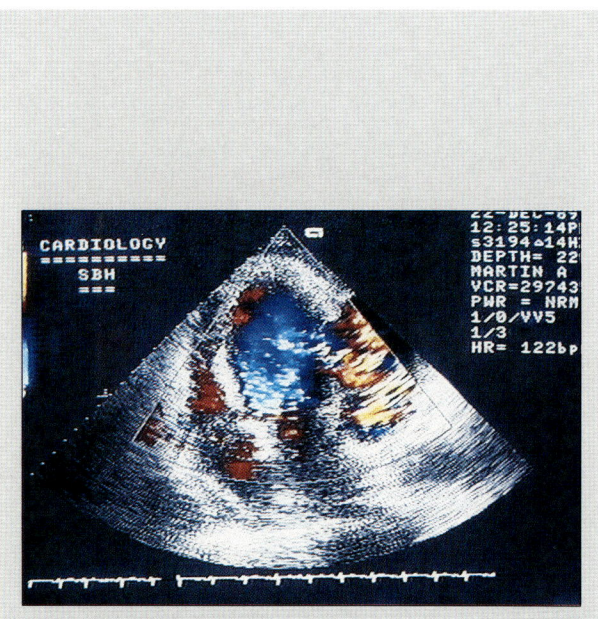

Figure 138 Same patient as in Figures 136 and 137 at end-diastole. The persistence of signal outside the rupture is seen

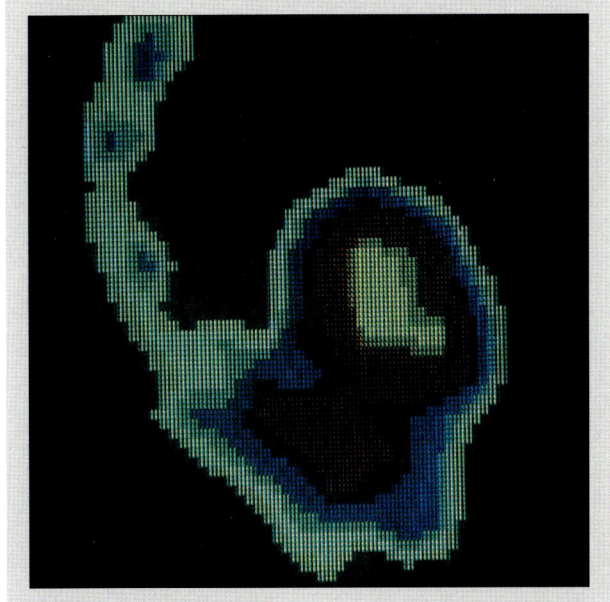

Figure 139 Frame from a first-pass radionuclide angiogram at end-diastole showing a large 'false' aneurysmal cavity attached to the anterior wall of the left ventricle

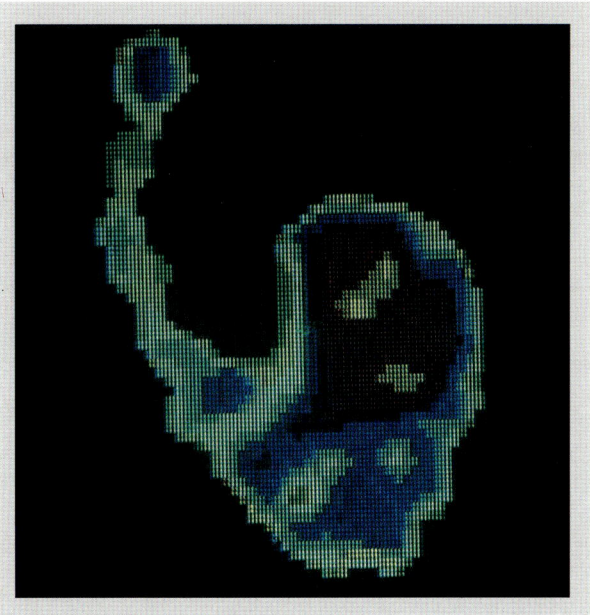

Figure 140 Same patient as in Figure 139 at end-systole. The main ventricle is now virtually empty of counts. The large ball of counts in red and yellow is blood in the aneurysmal sac

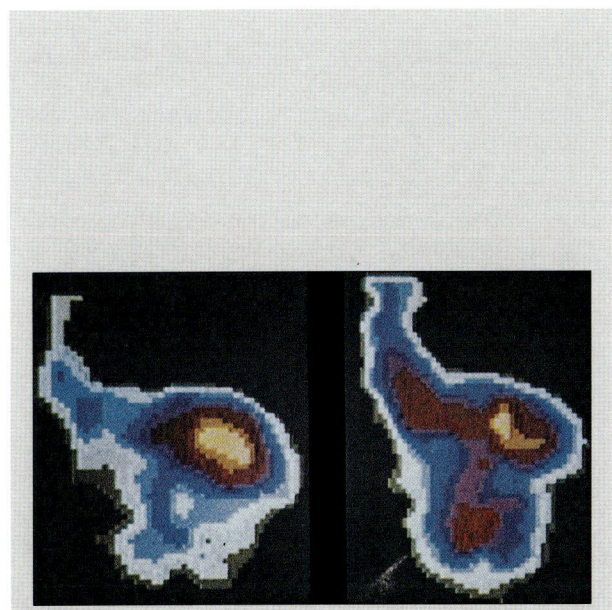

Figure 141 End-diastolic (left) and end-systolic (right) frames from a first-pass radionuclide angiogram showing a false left ventricular aneurysm inferiorly. The end-systolic image shows counts streaming through the narrow neck of the aneurysm into the sac. (Reprinted by permission from *Journal of Nuclear Medicine*, 1979, **20**, 851–4)

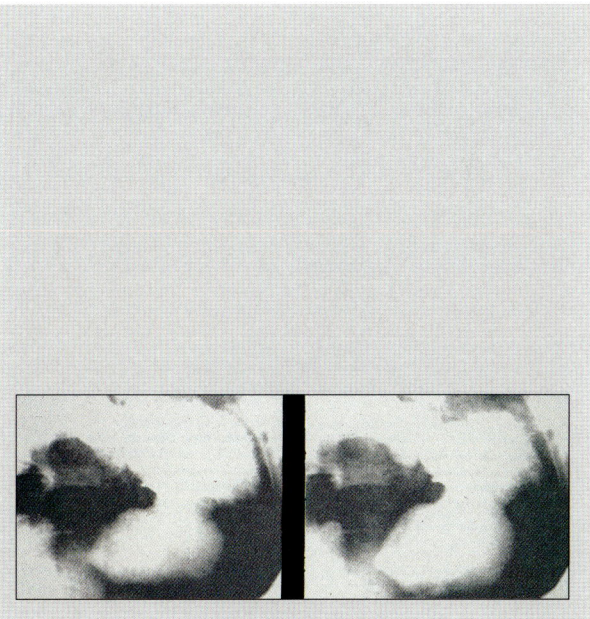

Figure 142 Contrast left ventriculogram from the same patient as in Figure 141 showing aneurysmal sac at end-diastole and end-systole. Note the expansion of the sac at end-systole. (Reprinted by permission from *Journal of Nuclear Medicine*, 1979, **20**, 851–4)

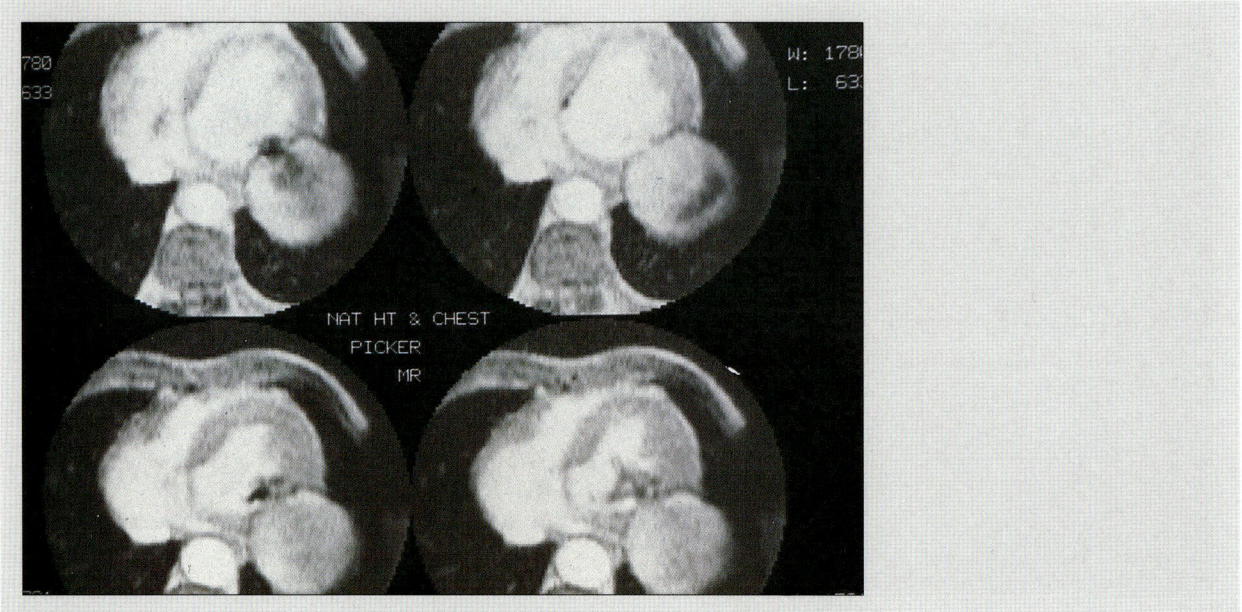

Figure 143 Four frames of a cine gradient echo acquisition from a magnetic resonance image in a patient with a recent infarction and a mass found incidentally on chest X-ray. The magnetic resonance images show it to be a false aneurysm. The top two images are systolic frames showing a jet of turbulent blood as loss of signal passing from the ventricle into the aneurysm. The lower two frames are diastolic showing the jet of turbulent flow from the aneurysm back into the ventricle

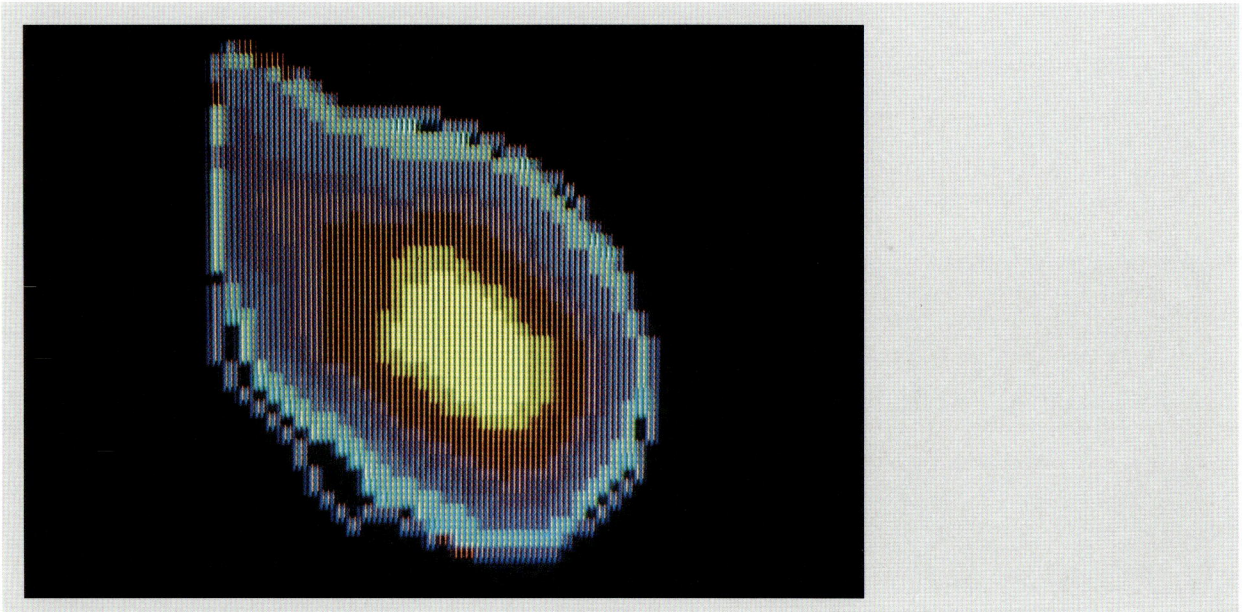

Figure 144 End-systolic frame with end-diastolic perimeter from a first-pass radionuclide angiogram of a patient with recurrent ventricular tachycardia and fibrillation. The measured ejection fraction was 7%

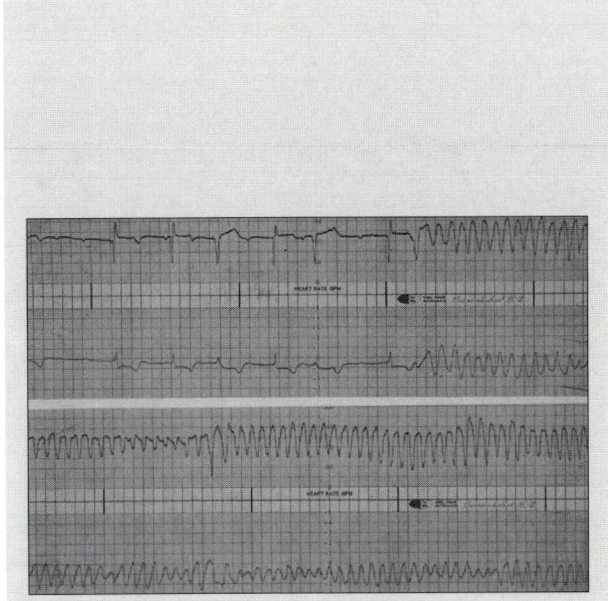

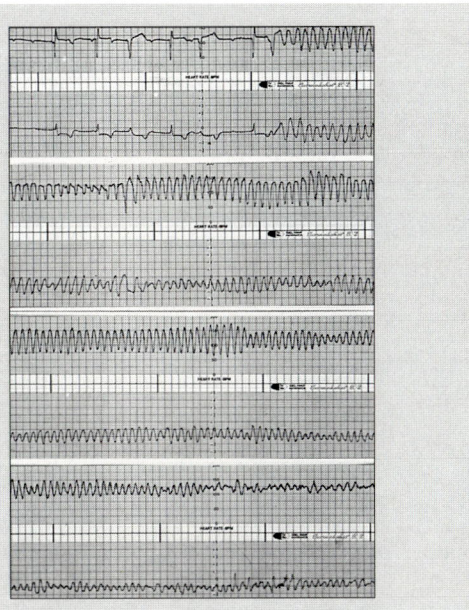

Figure 145 A strip from a Holter monitor of a patient with poor left ventricular function 12 days after myocardial infarction. The recording was taken in hospital. The top two panels are simultaneous and show an episode of complete heart block and then an R on T ectopic which promotes ventricular tachycardia and fibrillation. The patient suffered an in-hospital cardiac arrest and was defibrillated. This is known as secondary ventricular fibrillation

Figure 146 Fatal ventricular fibrillation in a patient 3 months after myocardial infarction being monitored on a Holter monitor out of hospital

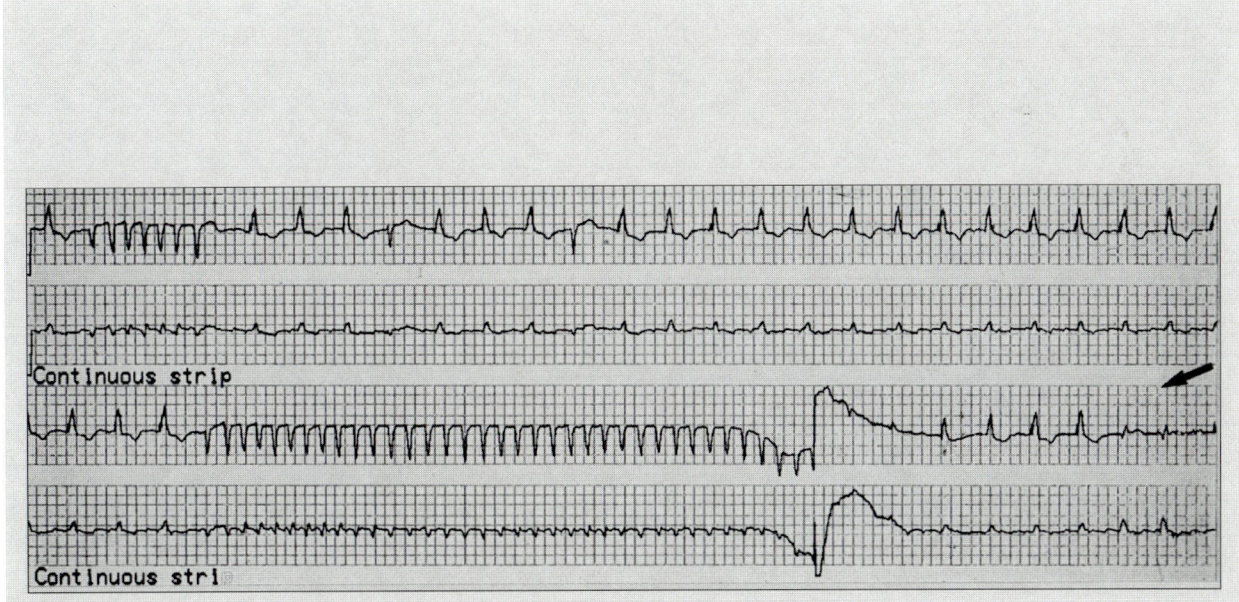

Figure 147 Continuous strip from a Holter monitor. The top two panels show an episode of non-sustained ventricular tachycardia followed by sinus rhythm. The bottom two panels show a sustained episode of ventricular tachycardia which was restored to sinus rhythm by the automatic delivery of a shock from an automatic implantable cardioverter defibrillator. Sinus rhythm recommences where the arrow marks

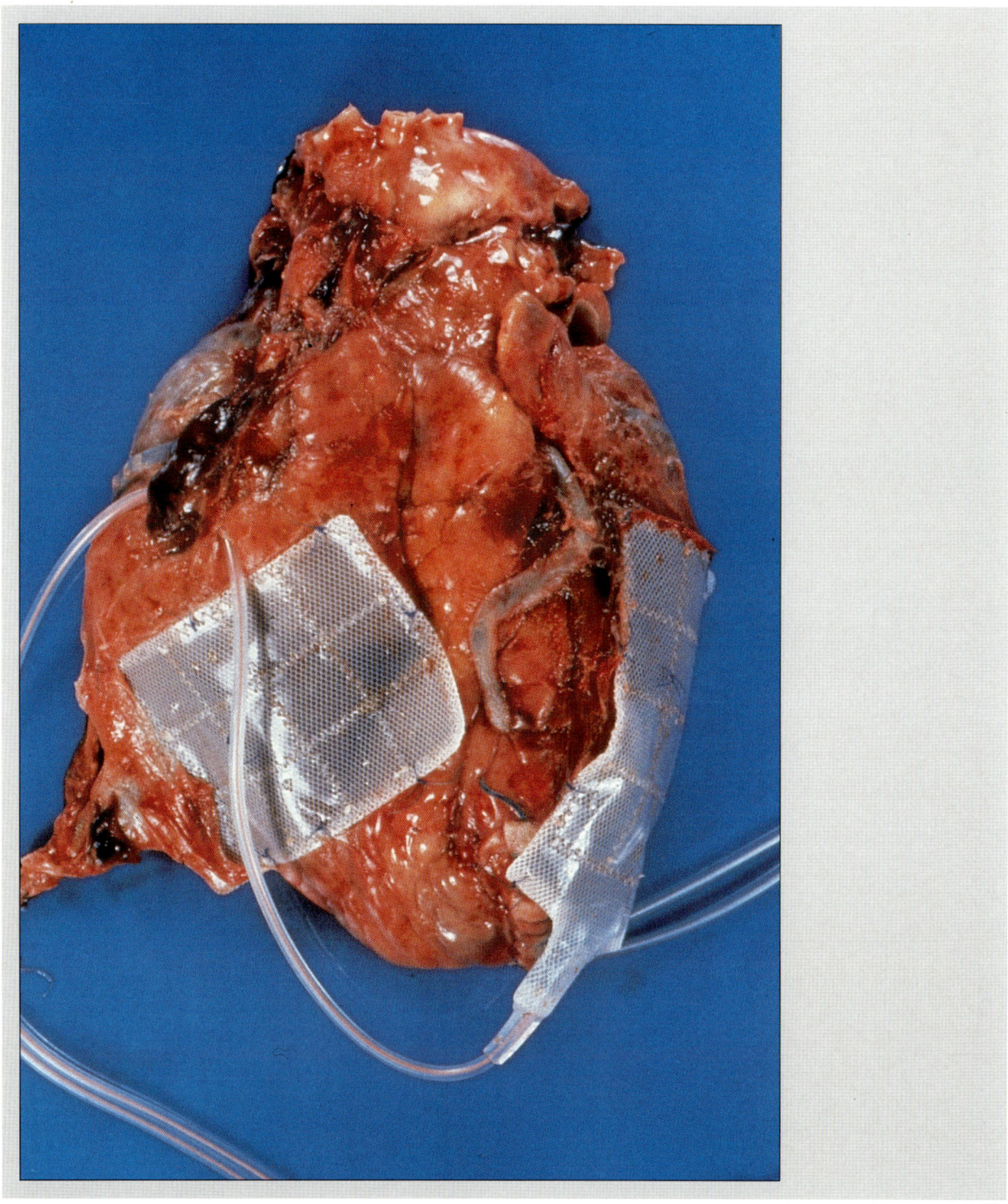

Figure 148 Explanted heart at postmortem showing the placement of the defibrillator patches of the automatic implantable cardioverter defibrillator

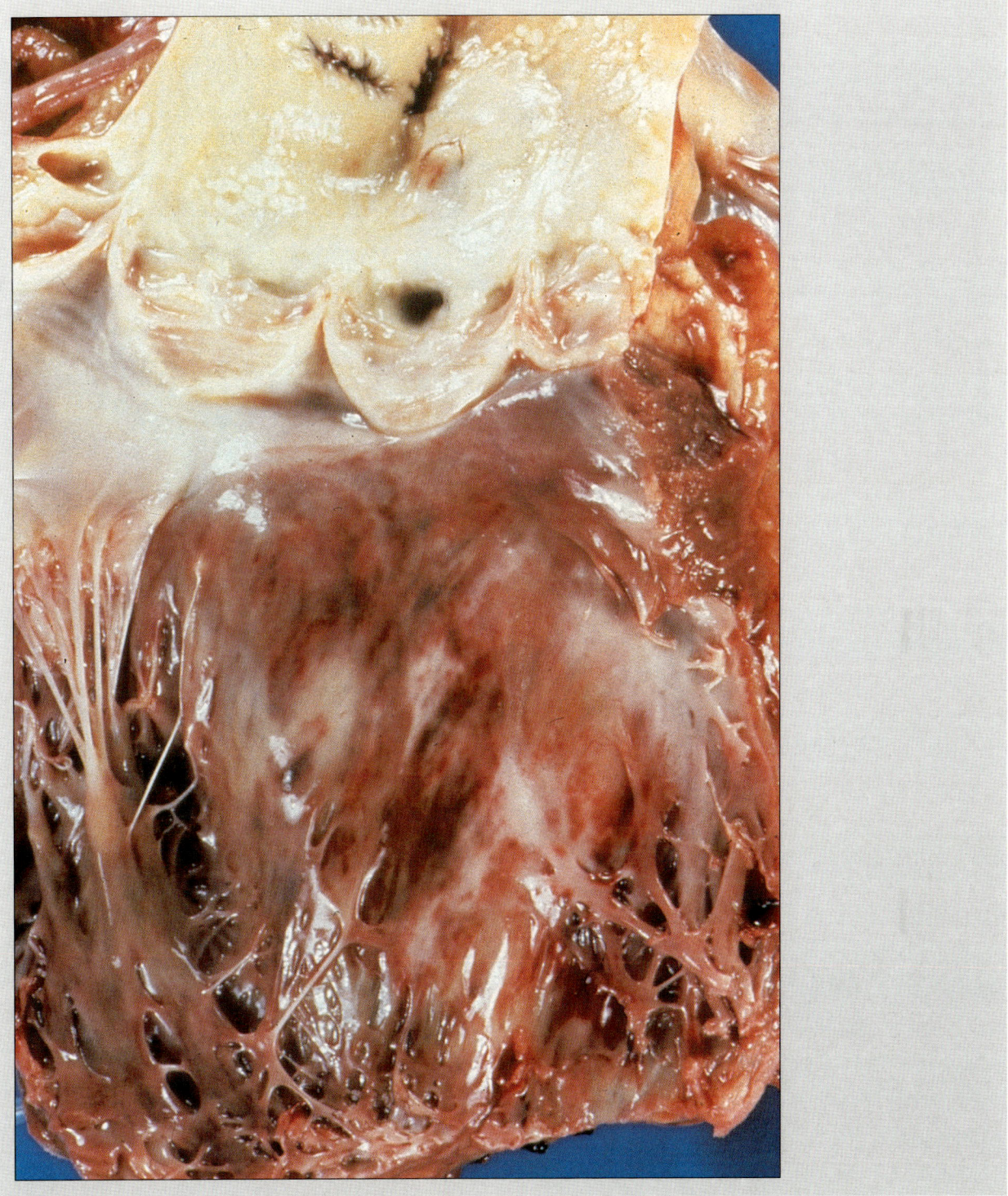

Figure 149 Postmortem heart showing the mottled, multiple hemorrhagic appearance of an infarct that was the focus for intractable ventricular tachycardia

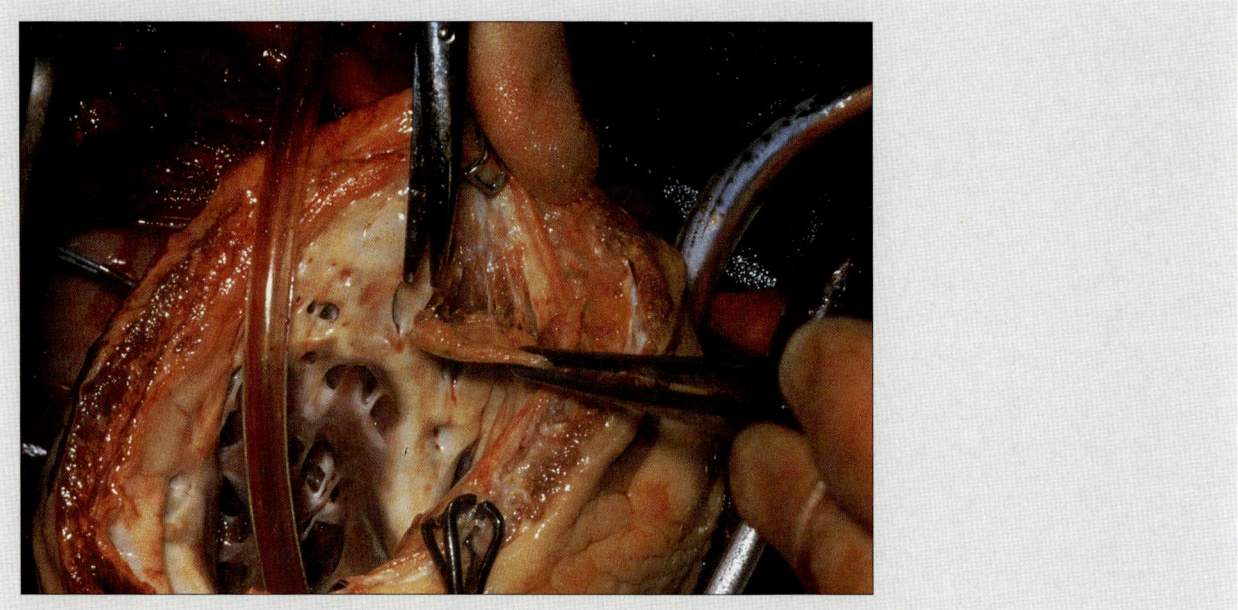

Figure 150 Resection of scarred endocardium being carried out surgically for ventricular tachycardia focus

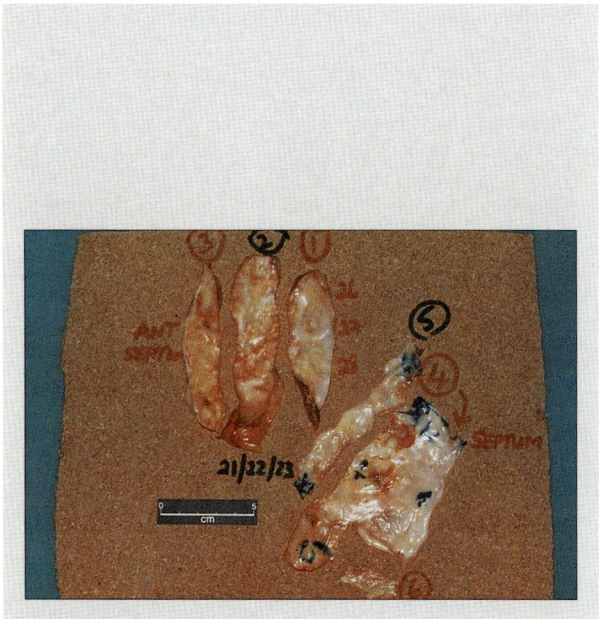

Figure 151 Samples of scarred endocardium resected surgically from a patient with myocardial infarction and ventricular tachycardia

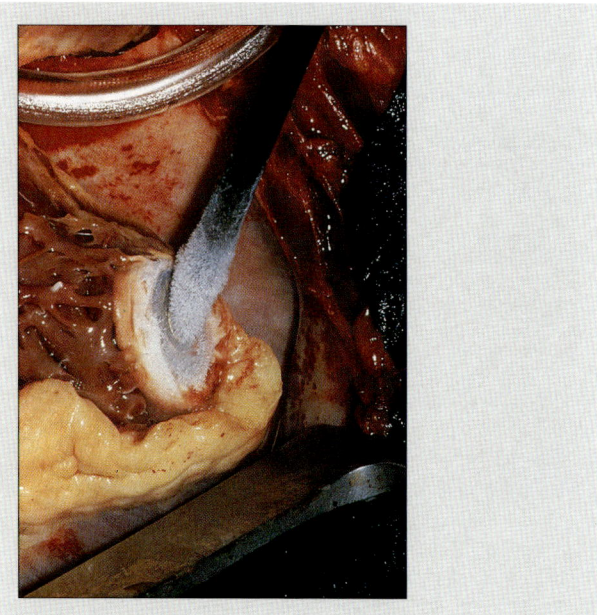

Figure 152 Cryoablation of ventricular tachycardia focus at operation

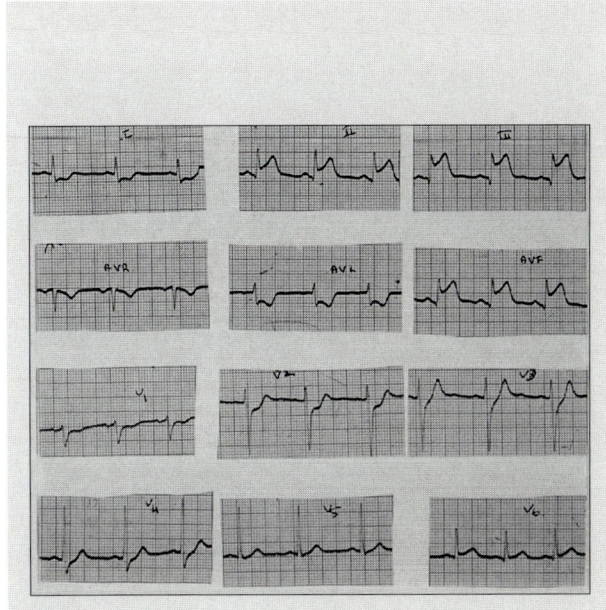

Figure 153 12-lead ECG from a patient with a 2-hour history of central crushing chest pain, showing acute inferior infarction changes with ST elevation in leads II, III and AVF

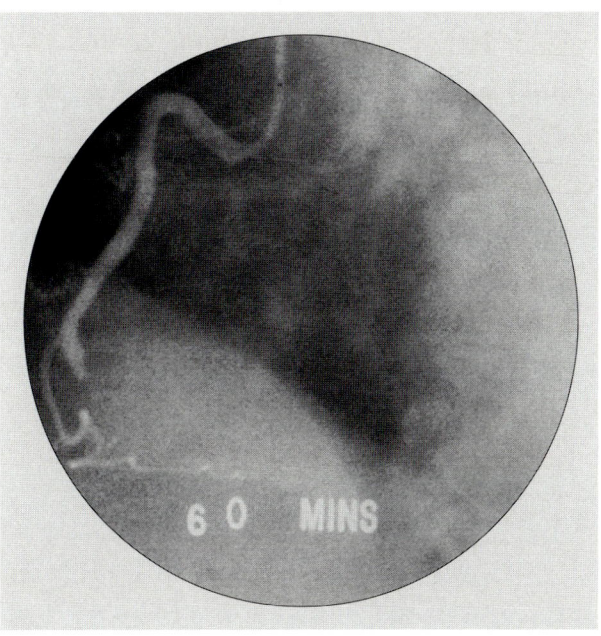

Figure 154 Selective right coronary arteriogram 60 min into an infusion of tissue plasminogen activator (t-PA) in the same patient as in Figure 153. The artery is occluded just above the crux

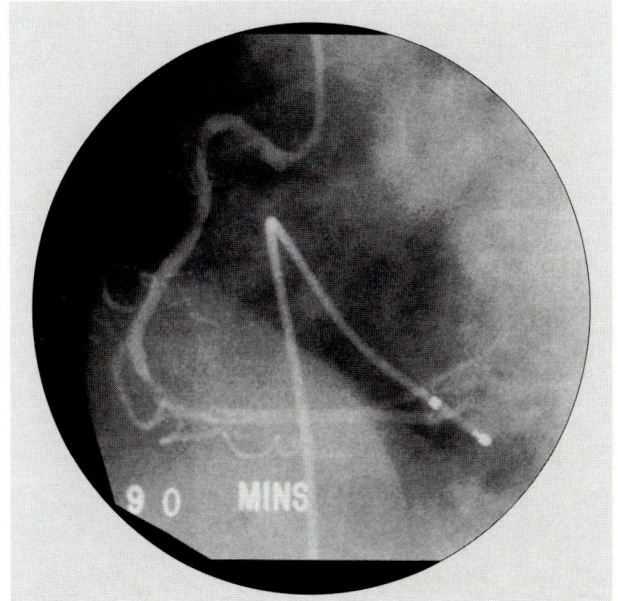

Figure 155 Selective right coronary arteriogram 90 min into the infusion of t-PA in the same patient as in Figures 153 and 154 showing restoration of patency into the distal right coronary artery and posterior descending artery although there is still some haziness at the site of the previous occlusion which indicates some residual thrombus

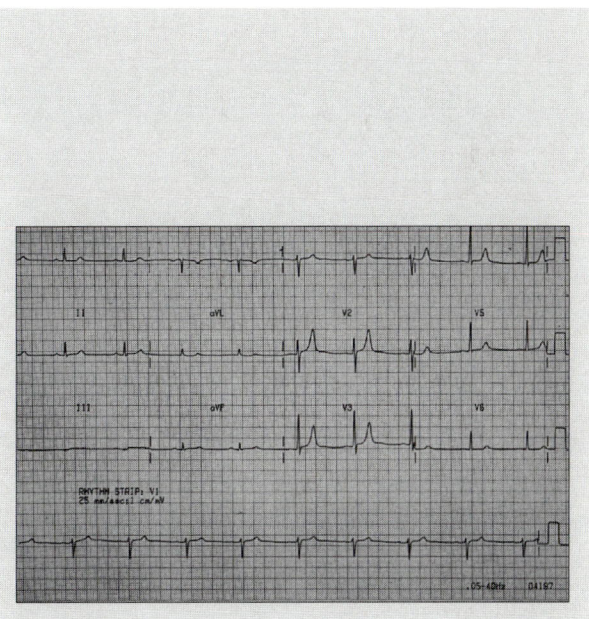

Figure 156 12-lead electrocardiogram following the completion of the t-PA infusion in the same patient as in Figures 153–155 showing total resolution of the inferior changes with no Q waves

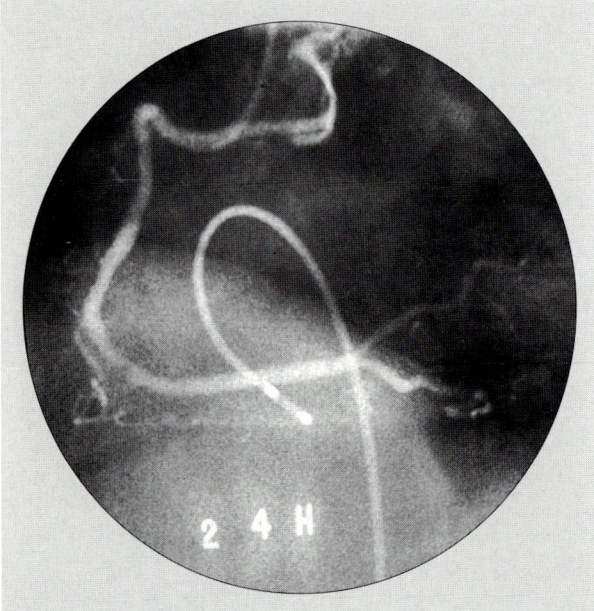

Figure 157 Selective right coronary angiogram of the same patient as in Figures 153–156 24 hours later. There is still a slight hazy filling defect at the site of the previous occlusion. This is less than before and there does not appear to be any significant hold-up of flow into the distal vessel. The patient had been maintained on heparin for the 24 hours after the completion of t-PA infusion

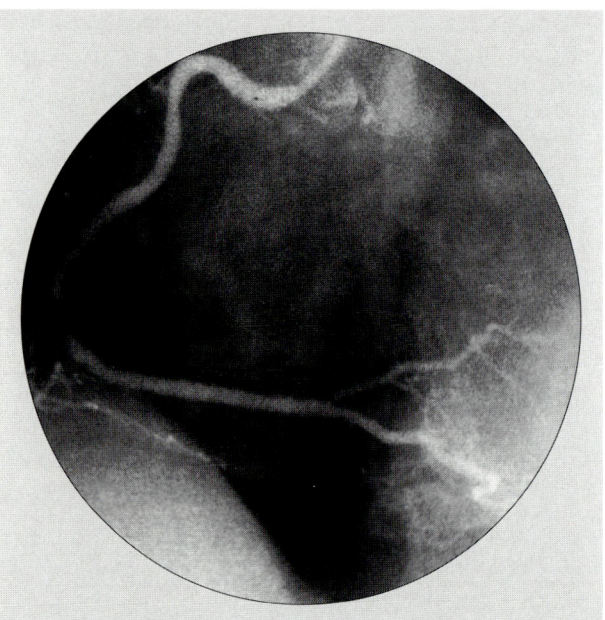

Figure 158 Selective right coronary arteriogram of the same patient as in Figures 153–157 3½ months later when she returned with angina pectoris after 150 meters exertion. Note that there has been remodelling at the site of the occlusion but there is now a significant stenosis in the right coronary artery at the site of the crux without any obvious residual thrombus

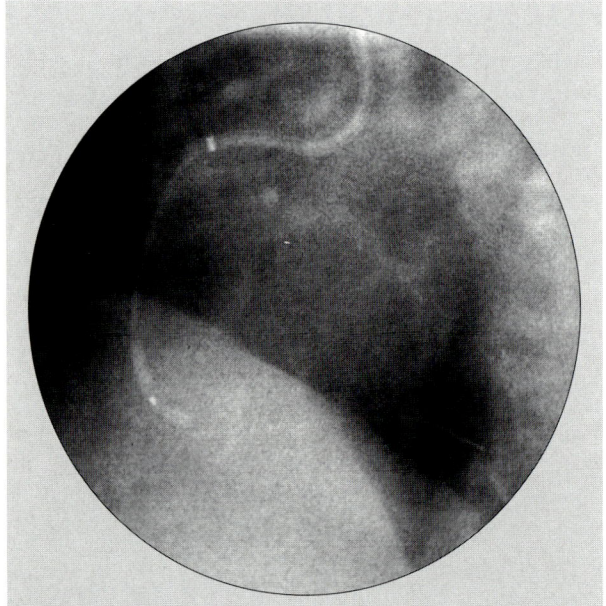

Figure 159 Angioplasty balloon being inflated over the right coronary stenosis in the same patient as in Figures 153–158. The tip of the guidewire is clearly seen anchored in the distal vessel

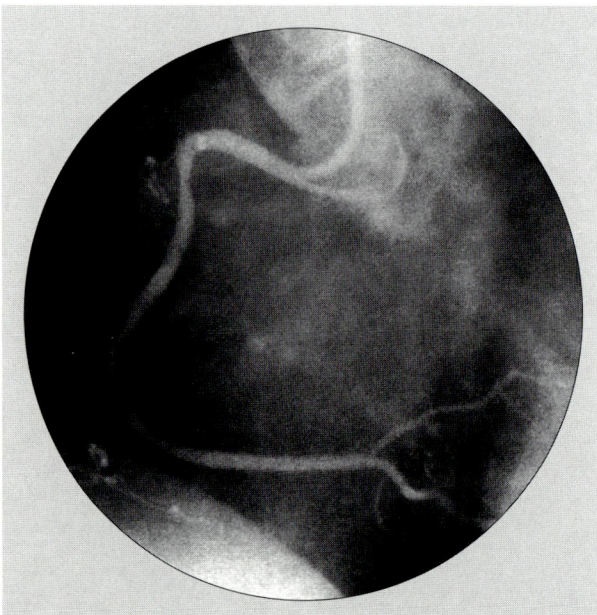

Figure 160 Final right coronary angiogram after successful angioplasty showing no residual stenosis and excellent antegrade flow in the same patient as in Figures 153–159

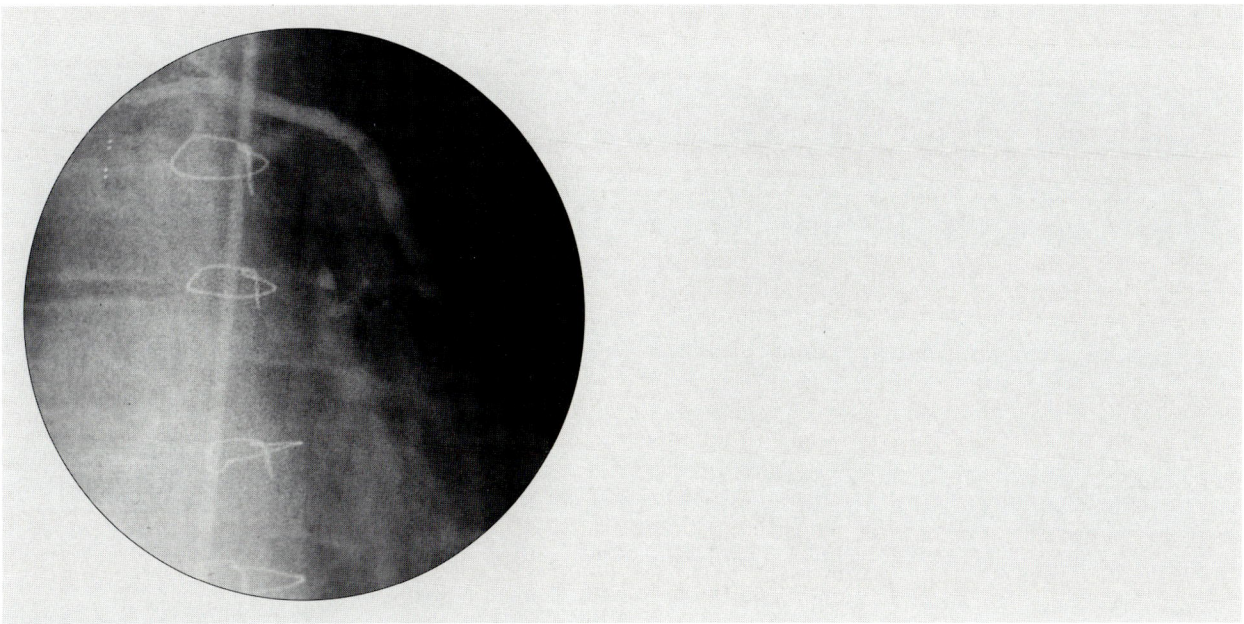

Figure 161 Selective injection into aorta to circumflex saphenous vein graft in a patient presenting with unstable angina 4 years after successful vein graft surgery. A large filling defect consisting of thrombus is seen in the body of the graft

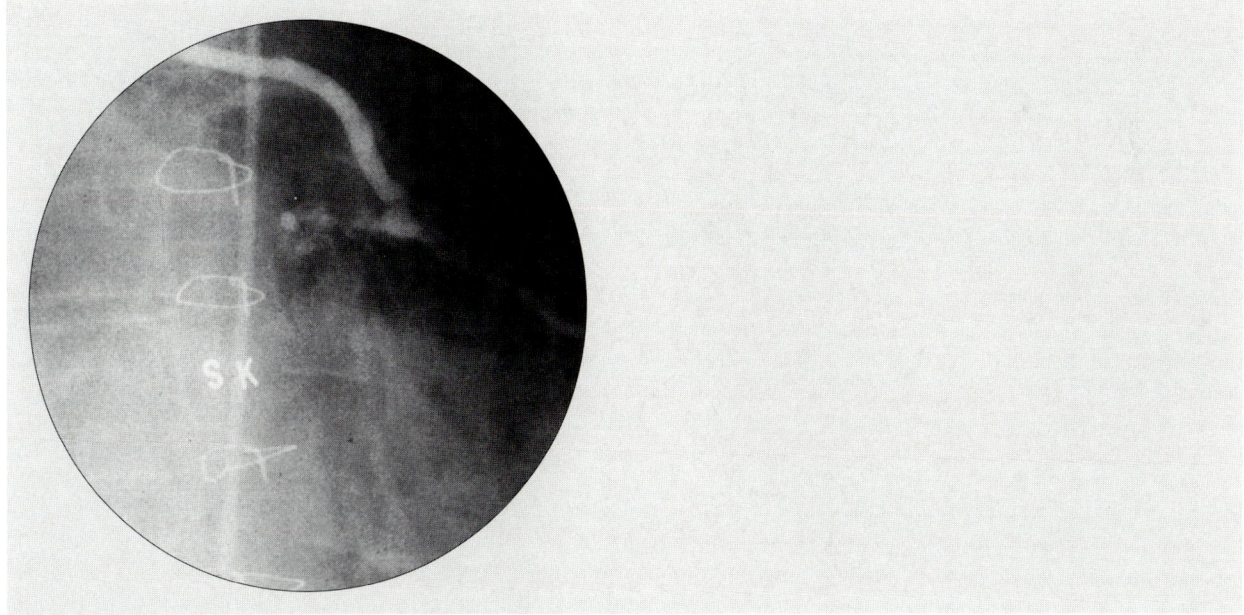

Figure 162 Same patient as in Figure 161 after infusion of 600 000 units of streptokinase into the vein graft over a 40-min period. The filling defect due to clot is no longer seen and there is now run-off into a patent but heavily diseased circumflex marginal artery

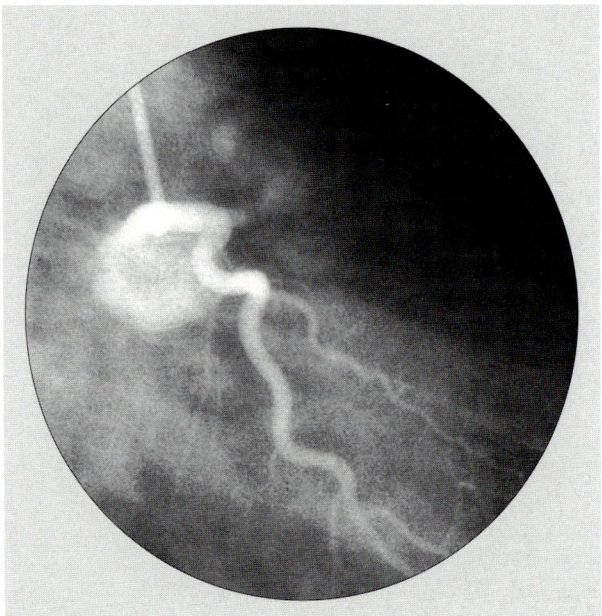

Figure 163 Selective left coronary angiogram showing a proximal and abrupt occlusion of the left anterior descending artery in a patient in whom thrombolytic therapy was contraindicated. The circumflex perfuses normally but there is no antegrade filling of the distal left anterior descending artery

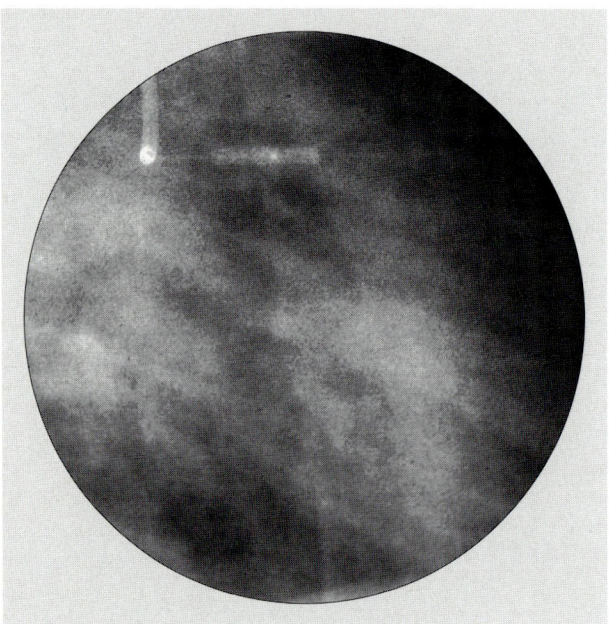

Figure 164 A primary angioplasty was carried out without thrombolytic therapy in the same patient as in Figure 163 within an hour of presentation to hospital. The guidewire is seen across the occluded left anterior descending artery with the balloon inflated

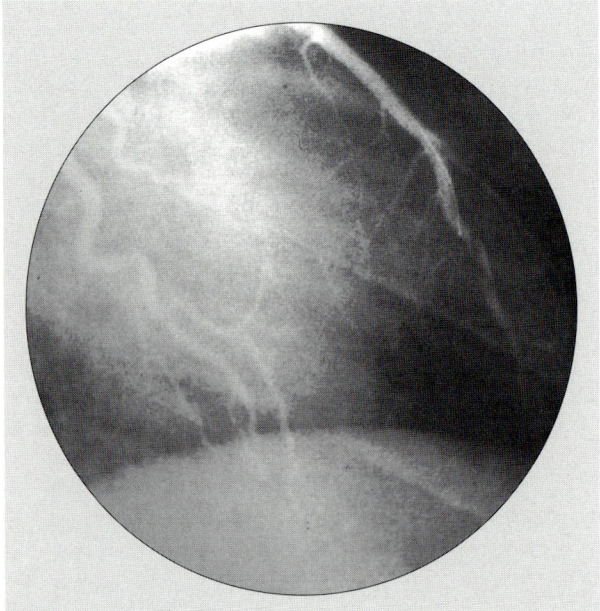

Figure 165 Selective angiogram of the left coronary artery in the same patient as in Figures 163 and 164 showing that the distal left anterior descending artery is now filling antegradely, although some clot has been displaced just beyond the tip of the guidewire, producing a filling defect in the middle portion of the vessel

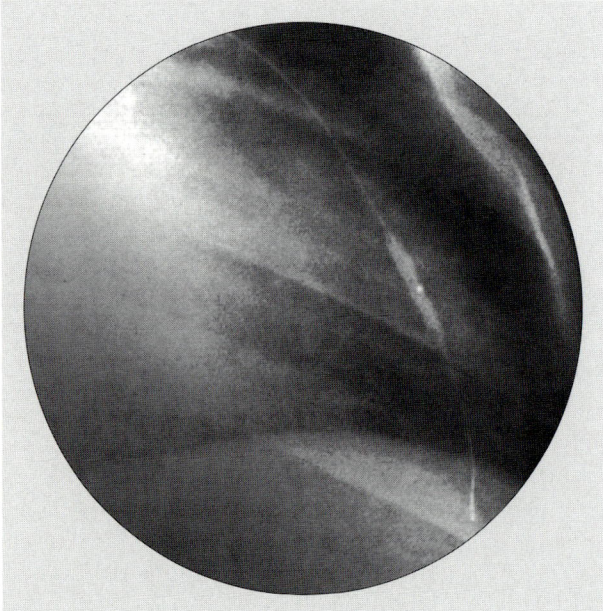

Figure 166 Further angioplasty carried out in the same patient as Figures 163–165 at the site of the displaced thrombus. The balloon is shown inflated

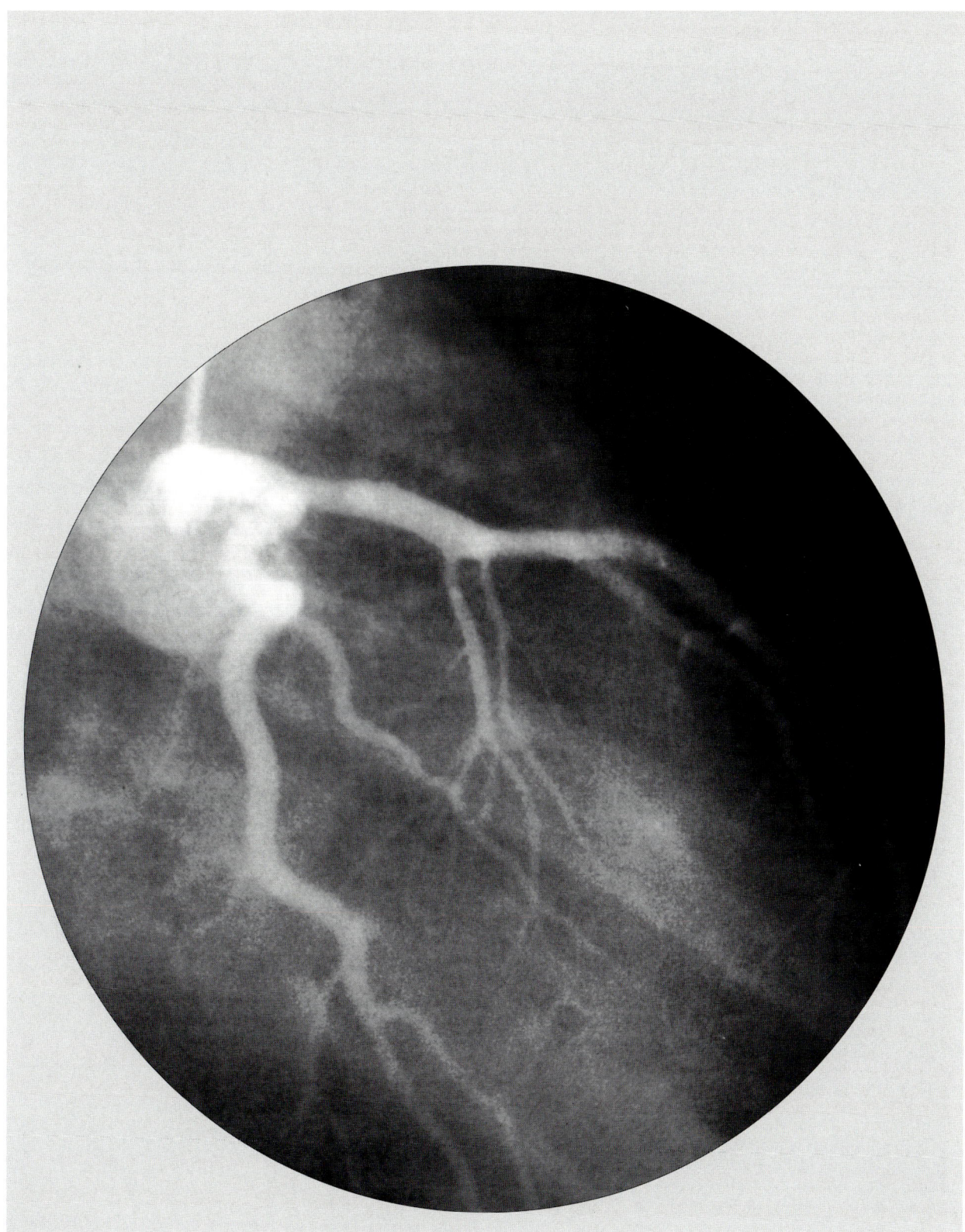

Figure 167 Final selective left coronary angiogram in the same patient as Figures 163–166 after complete recanalization of the left anterior descending artery with direct angioplasty. The diagonal branches and the septal perforators are also clearly seen

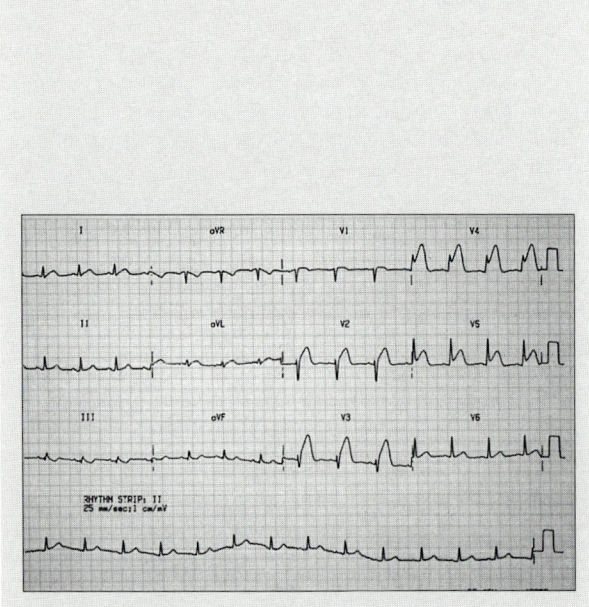

Figure 168 12-lead electrocardiogram showing acute ST segment elevation in leads V2–V5 with some hyperacute changes as well in leads I, AVL and V6 in a patient with prior bypass surgery in whom thrombolytic therapy was contraindicated

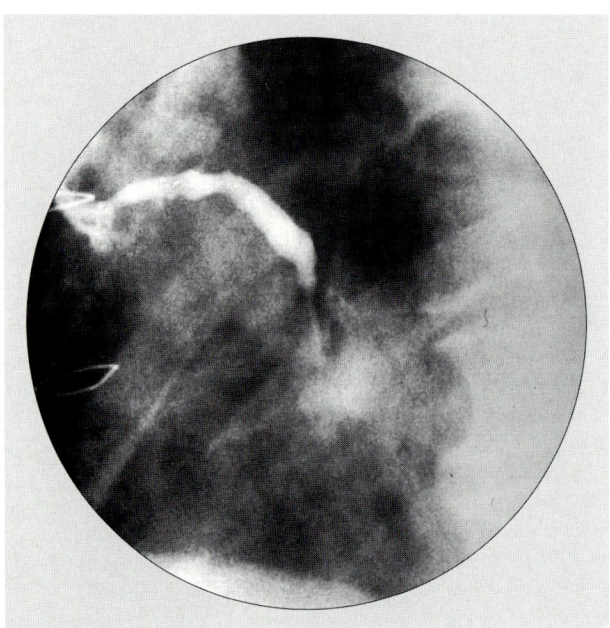

Figure 169 Selective injection into the ostium of the aorta to left anterior descending artery via the saphenous vein graft in the same patient as in Figure 169. The vein graft is rather irregular and shows signs of attrition, but there is a virtual complete occlusion at the site of the anastomosis of the vein graft into the native left anterior descending

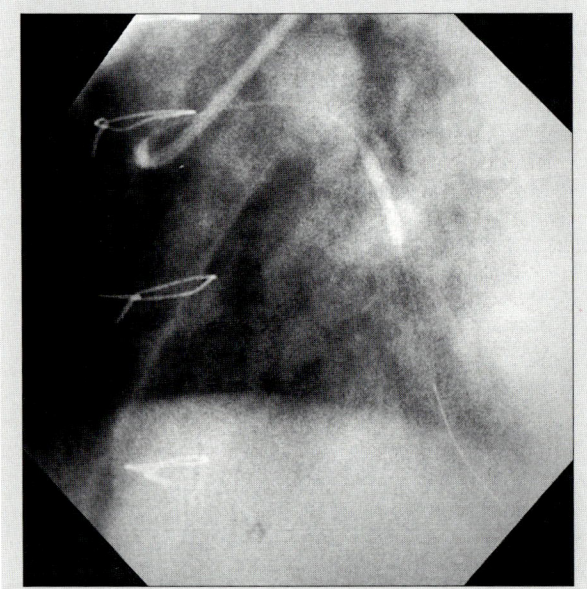

Figure 170 Direct angioplasty to the left anterior descending artery via the saphenous vein graft in the same patient as Figures 168 and 169. The guidewire is seen exiting from the guiding catheter passing through the vein and into the distal left anterior descending artery and the balloon is shown inflated at the site of the occlusion

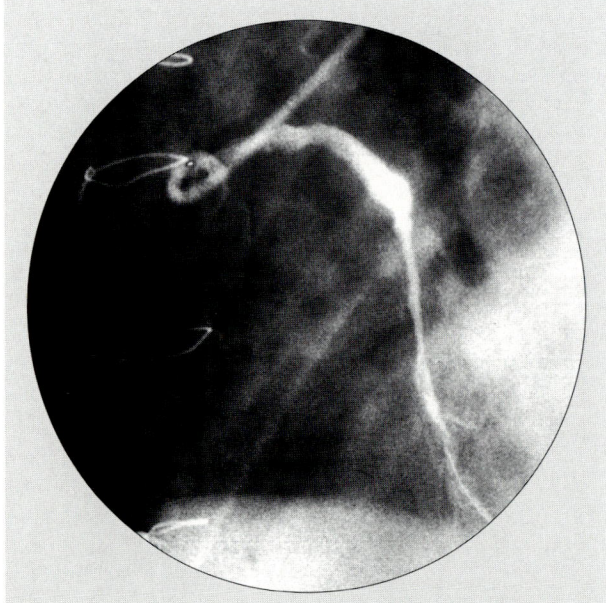

Figure 171 Final selective injection into aorta to left anterior descending artery saphenous vein graft after recanalization of the left anterior descending with angioplasty in the same patient as Figures 168–170. Note that there is now excellent run-off into a satisfactory distal left anterior descending

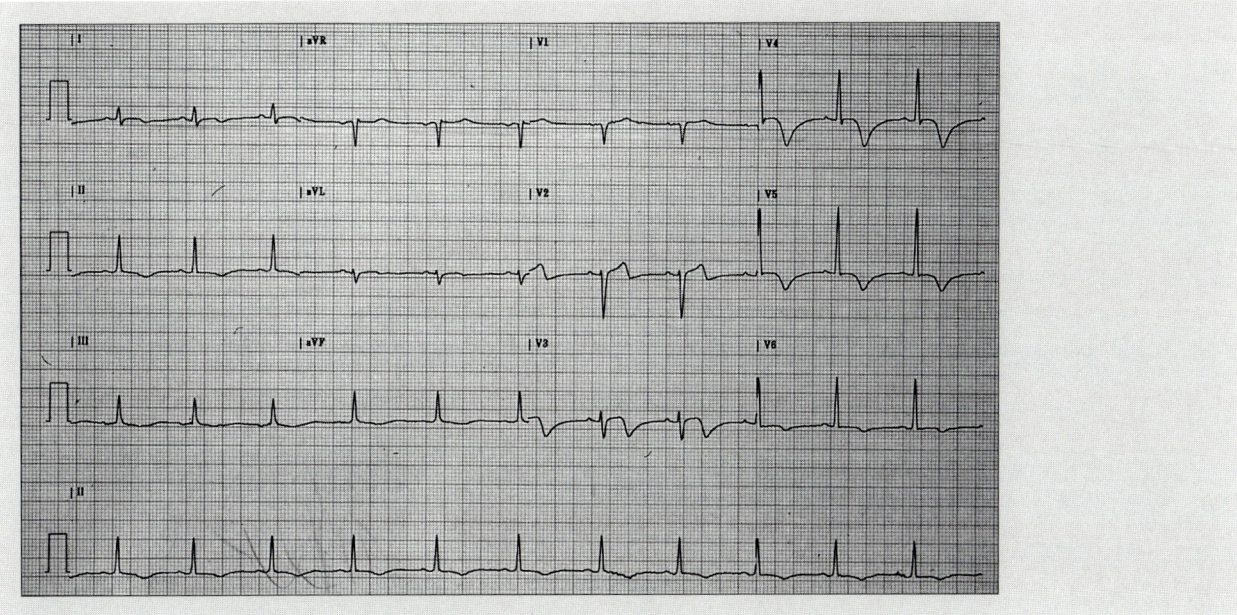

Figure 172 12-lead electrocardiogram in the same patient as in Figures 168–171 12 hours after successful direct angioplasty. The ST segments have returned to normal, there are no Q waves but there is T wave inversion from V2 to V5 and in I, II and V6

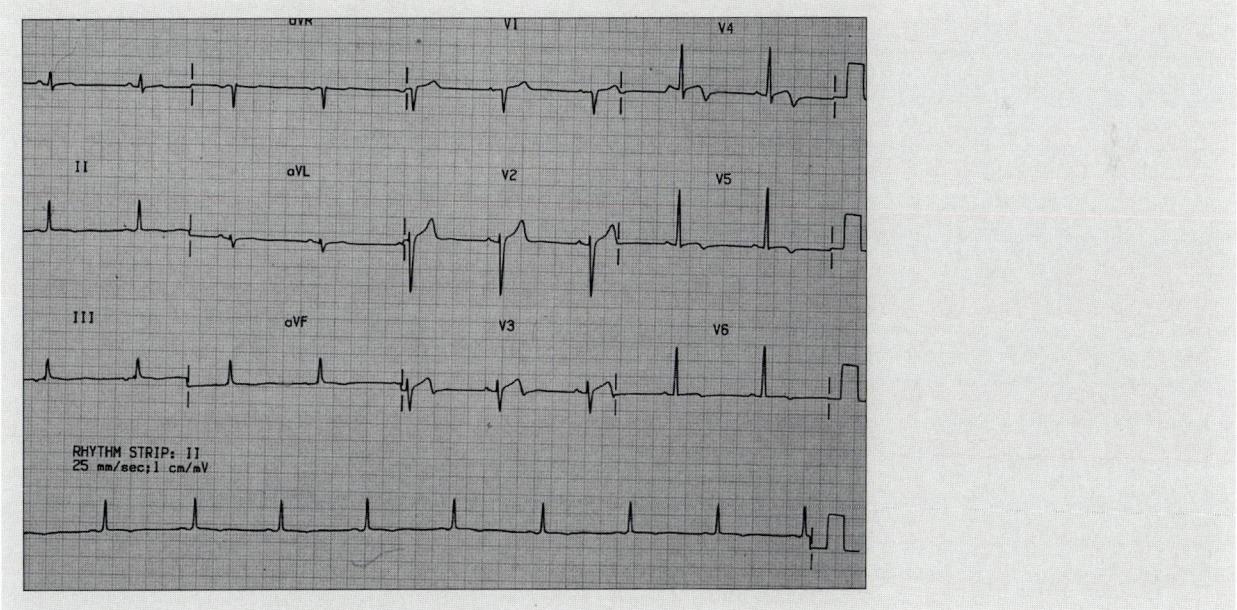

Figure 173 ECG from same patient as in Figures 168–172 1 week later showing further resolution of the ECG changes

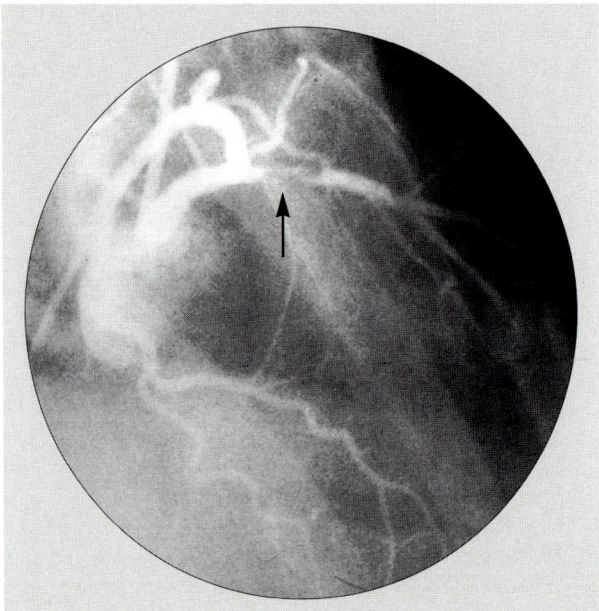

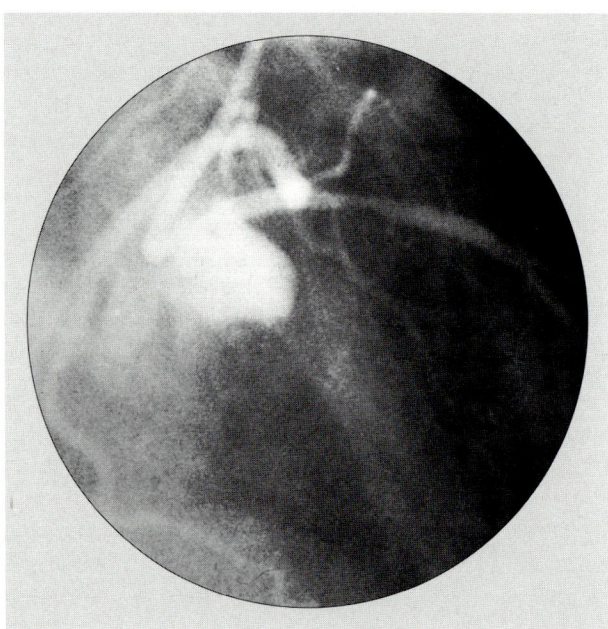

Figure 174 Selective left coronary angiogram in the cranial right anterior oblique projection showing a long, ragged proximal left anterior descending stenosis with some associated thrombus (arrowed). This was from a 75-year-old lady who presented with an anterior myocardial infarction and who received thrombolytic therapy but continued to experience prolonged postinfarction chest pain refractory to intravenous nitrates

Figure 175 Same patient as in Figure 174 after coronary angioplasty. There has been some improvement of the lesion, although the artery is still narrowed by significant stenosis and the patient continued to experience chest pain

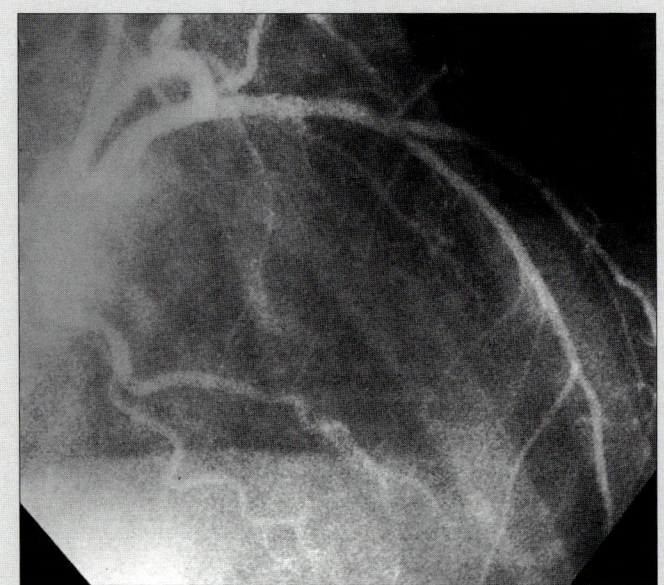

Figure 176 Same patient as in Figures 174 and 175 after implantation of a 3.5 mm balloon expandable intracoronary stent. The lumen of the artery now appears smooth with excellent antegrade flow; the patient's symptoms resolved

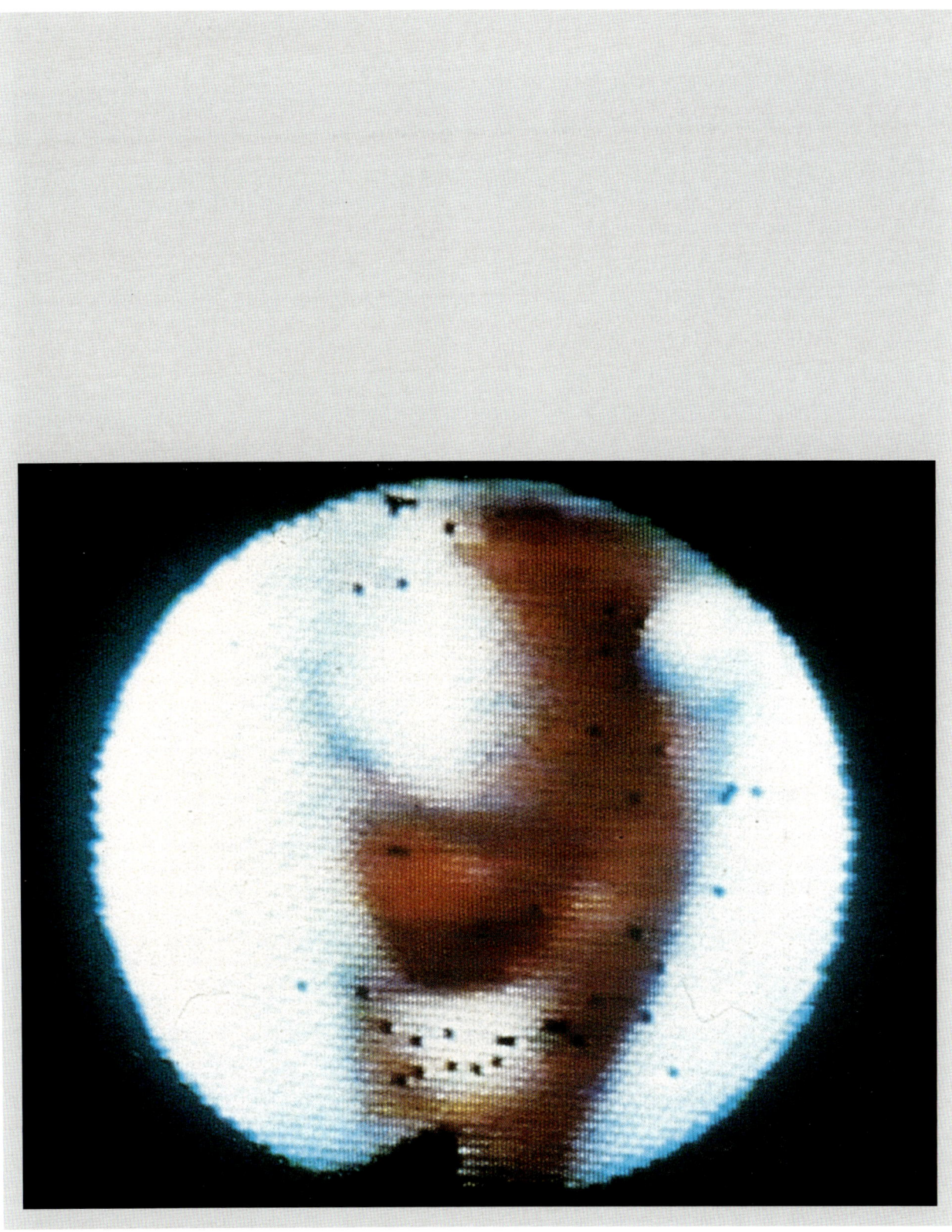

Figure 177 Angioscopic view of a patient with an abrupt occlusion of the right coronary artery. The endothelium of the coronary artery is shown in white but there is an obvious occlusive bright red thrombus obstructing the entire artery

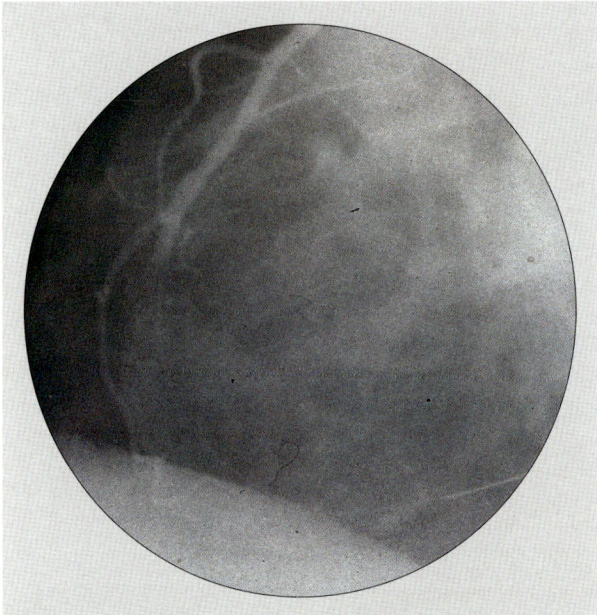

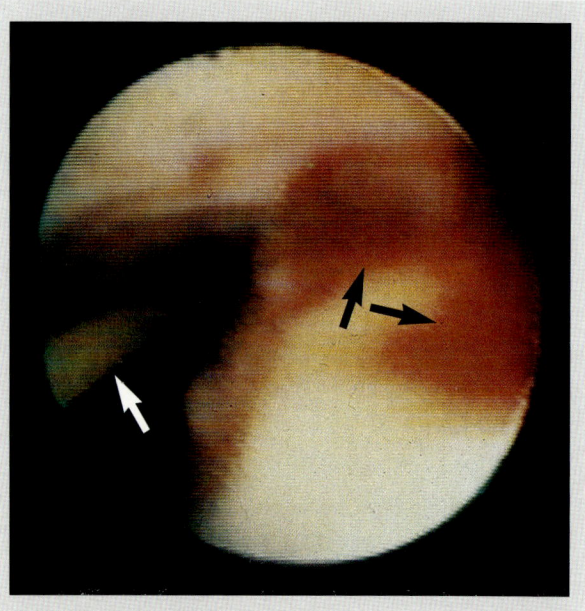

Figure 178 A frame from a coronary angiogram showing the site of an abrupt occlusion of the right coronary artery just beyond the right ventricular branch. A guidewire is seen passing through the occlusion anchored in the distal right coronary bed

Figure 179 Angioscopic view after recanalization of the lesion in Figure 178 with a guidewire and direct balloon angioplasty. The guidewire is seen passing distally and is shown on the angioscopy picture as a yellowish linear structure tapering distally (white arrow). A large amount of residual thrombus is seen subintimally after angioplasty. The thrombus is shown as a crescent-shaped red shadow (black arrows)

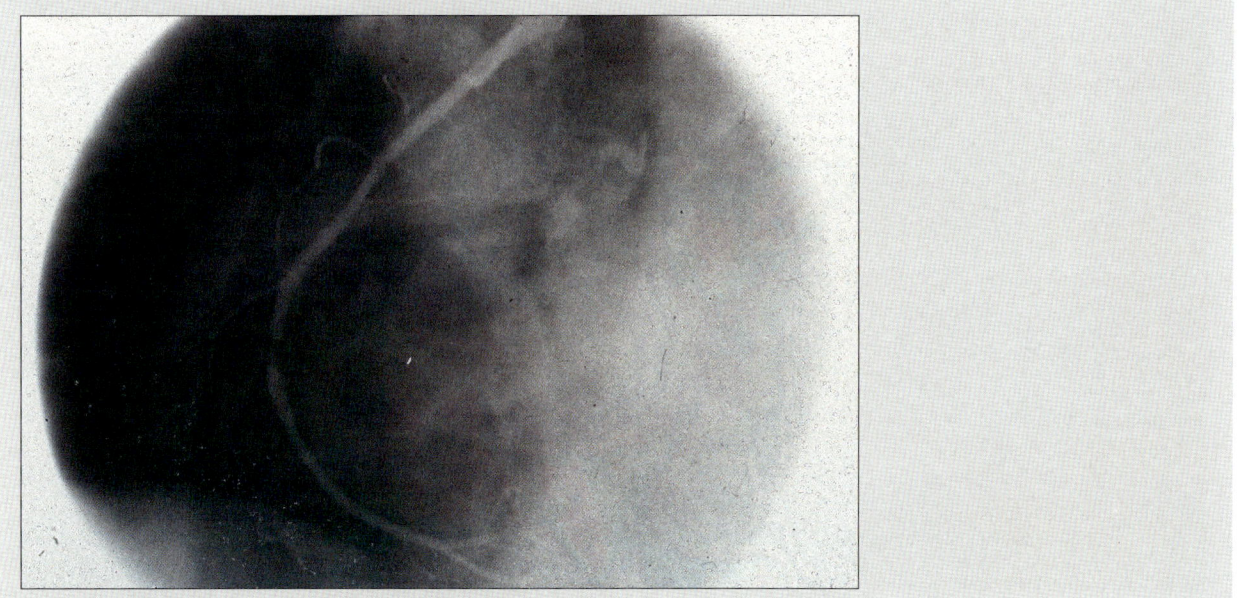

Figure 180 Coronary arteriogram from the same patient as in Figures 178 and 179 after recanalization. Note that the artery is widely patent but there is a tight stenosis just beyond the site of the occlusion, although the distal vessel opacifies well

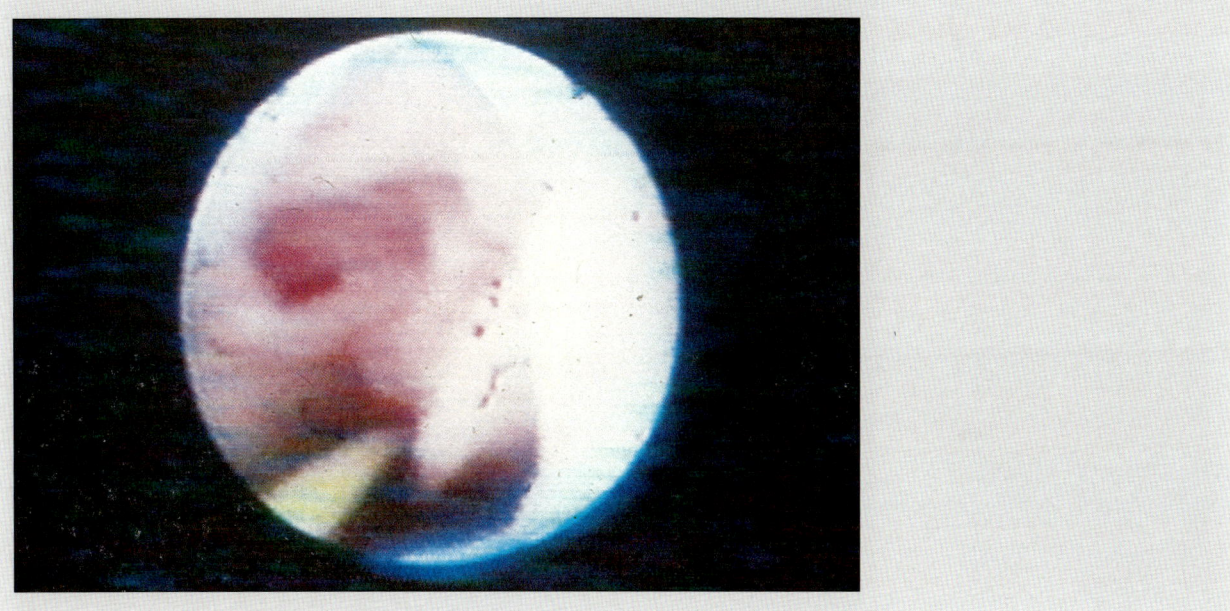

Figure 181 Angioscopic view of the right coronary stenosis demonstrated in Figure 180. Again the guidewire is seen at the bottom left-hand corner of the picture passing distally. There is a large amount of atheroma obstructing the lumen with some thrombus shown in red

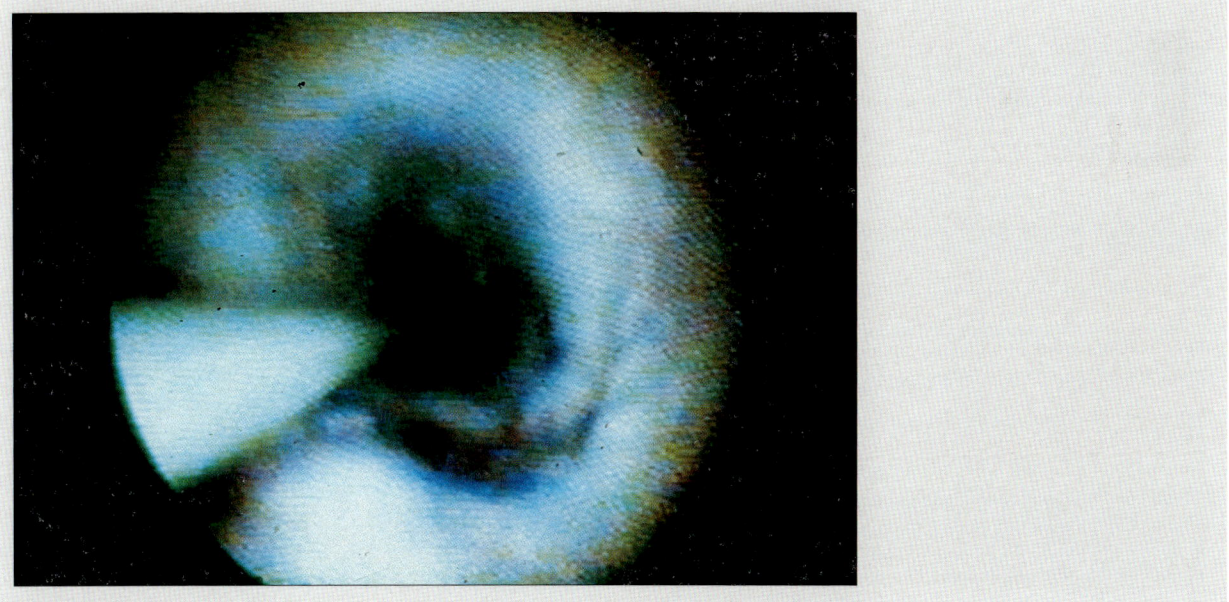

Figure 182 Angioscopic view of same lesion as in Figures 180 and 181 after successful angioplasty. The guidewire is shown this time as a whitish structure tapering distally; the patent lumen is shown in black but note the irregularity of the lumen and the residual thrombus subintimally in the lower wall of the artery. The intima still shows marked irregularity and there are some cracks in the plaque caused by the balloon

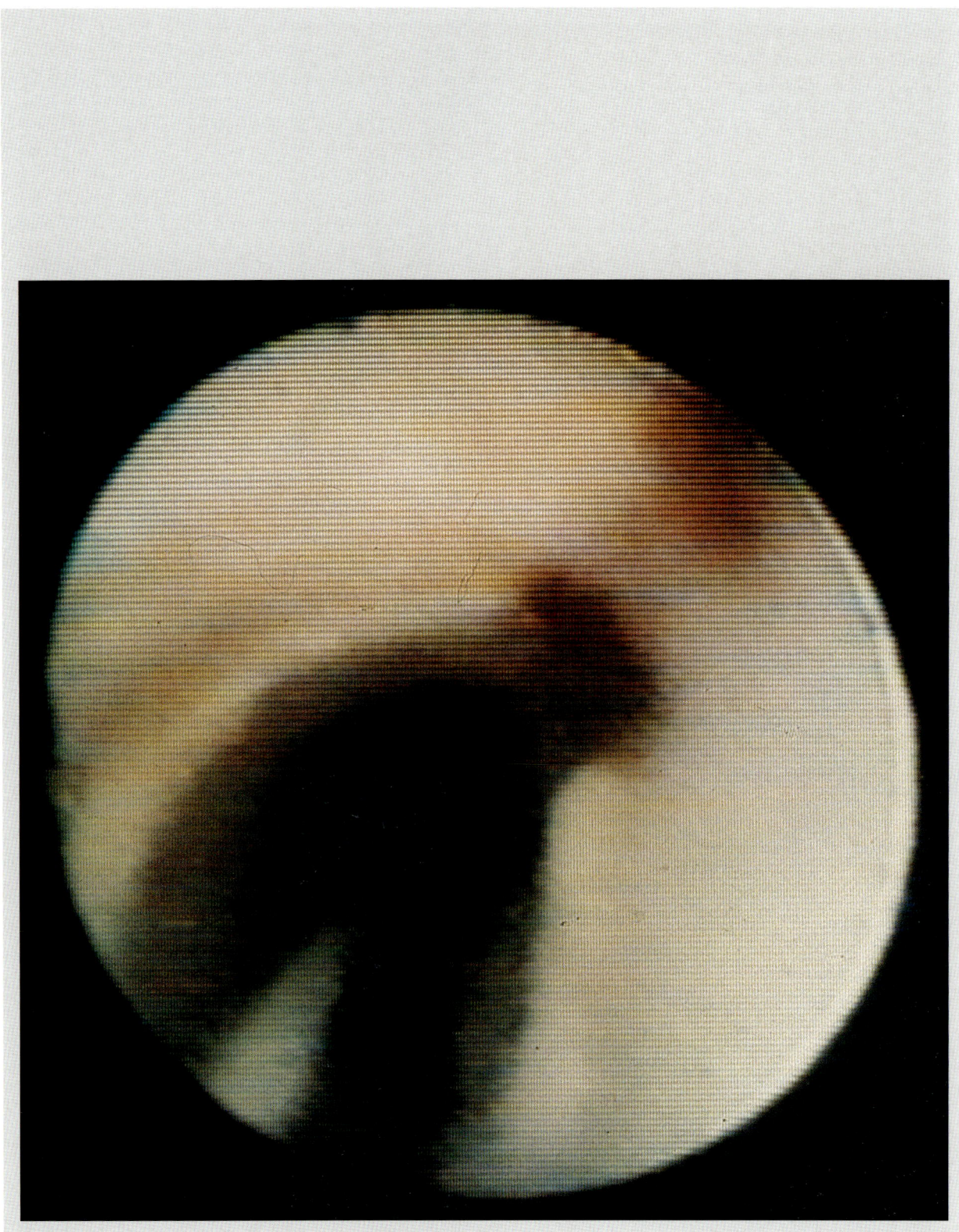

Figure 183 Angioscopic view of a vessel postangioplasty in a patient with unstable angina. The guidewire is again seen as a whitish structure passing linearly. Note that the lumen, shown in black, is quite large and regular with only a small flap in the right-hand side. There are, however, two areas of residual thrombus subintimally in the top right-hand corner of the picture

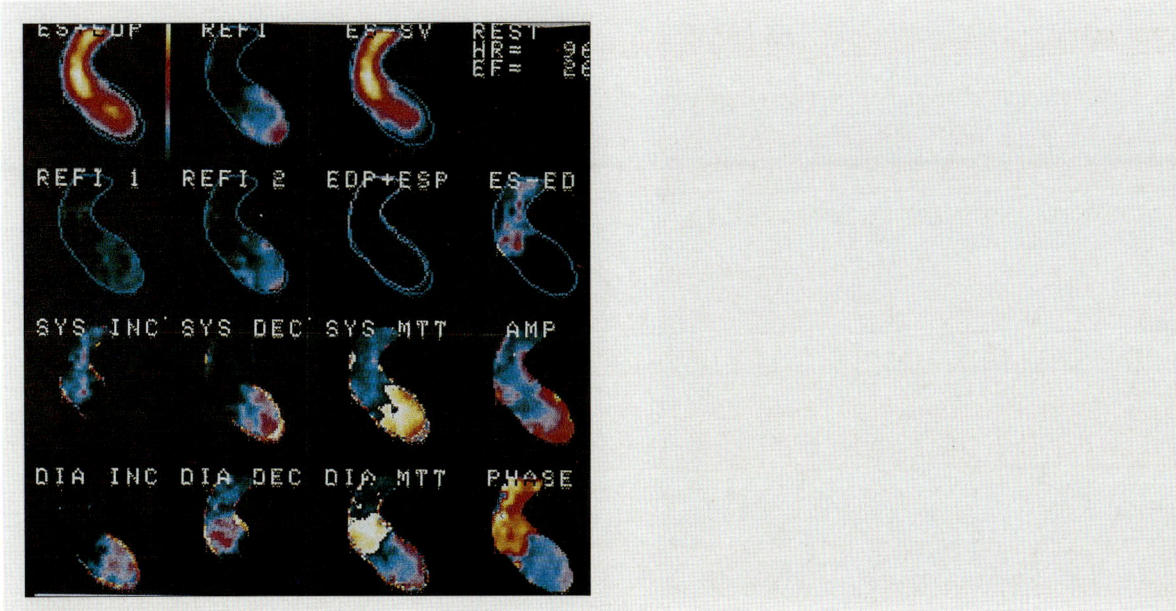

Figure 184 First-pass radionuclide angiogram taken 1 week after a patient presented with chest pain and marked anterior ST segment elevation. He received streptokinase with virtual normalization of the electrocardiogram. Note that the ejection fraction is reduced to 26% and the images show global left ventricular hypokinesis

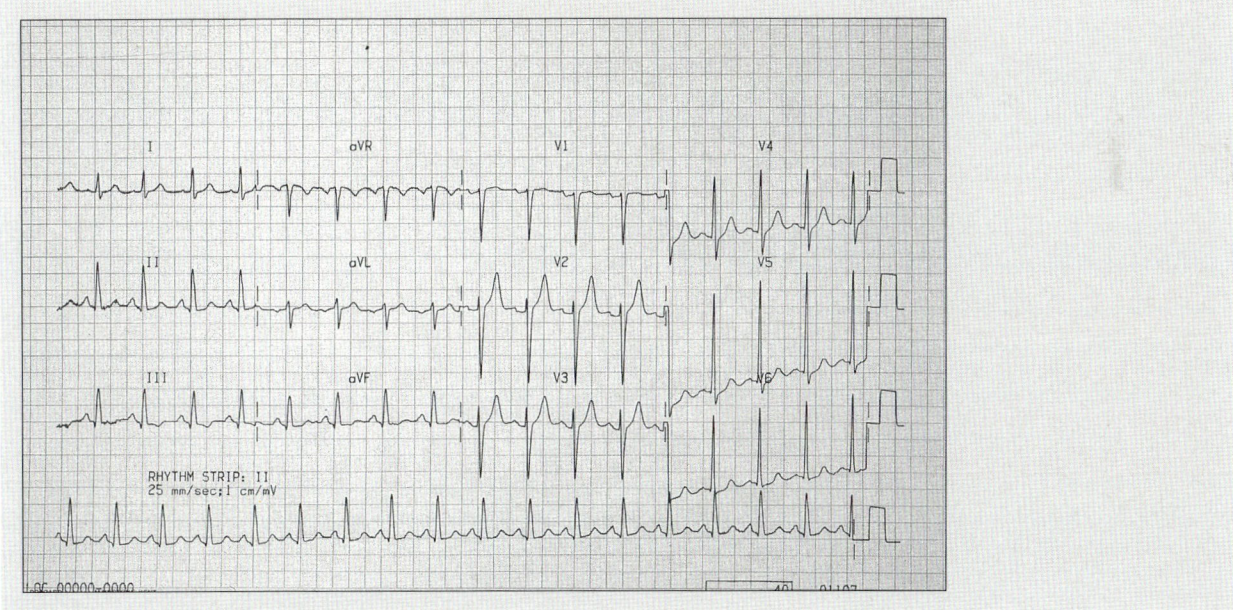

Figure 185 12-lead electrocardiogram from the same patient as in Figure 184 on the same day as the radionuclide study was obtained. There is some left ventricular hypertrophy on voltage criteria and some minor inferior changes. Otherwise the electrocardiogram does not show any evidence of infarction

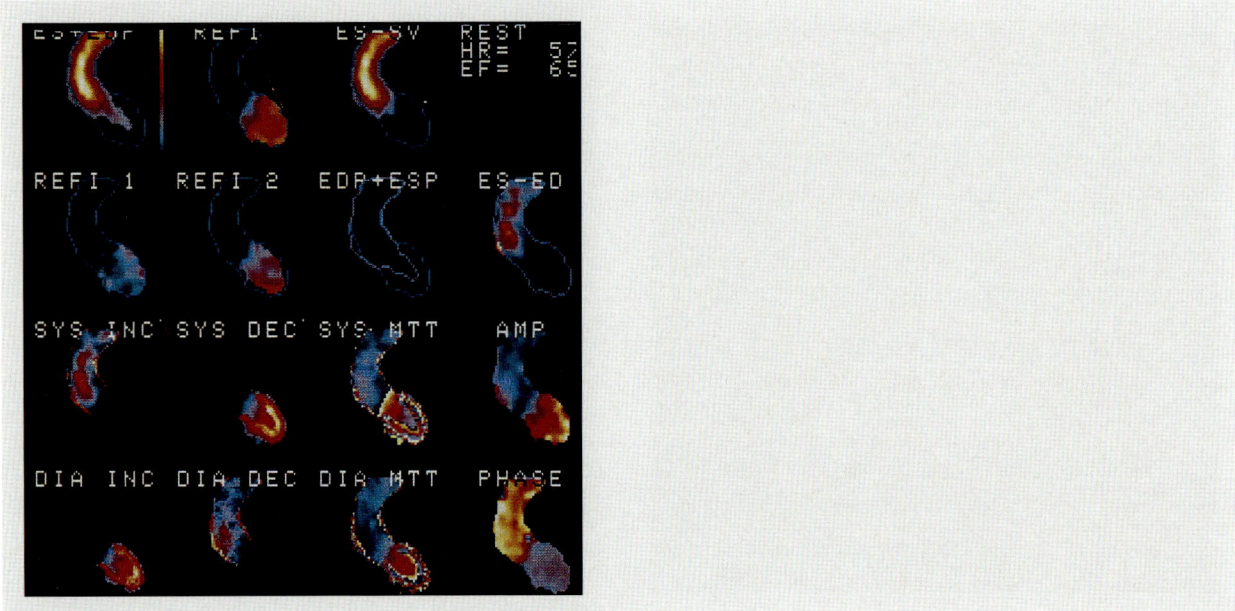

Figure 186 First-pass radionuclide angiogram in the same patient as in Figures 184 and 185 1 month later. Note that the ejection fraction has risen to 65% with normal wall motion globally. The initial radionuclide angiogram that showed global dysfunction was an example of 'stunning' which has spontaneously recovered

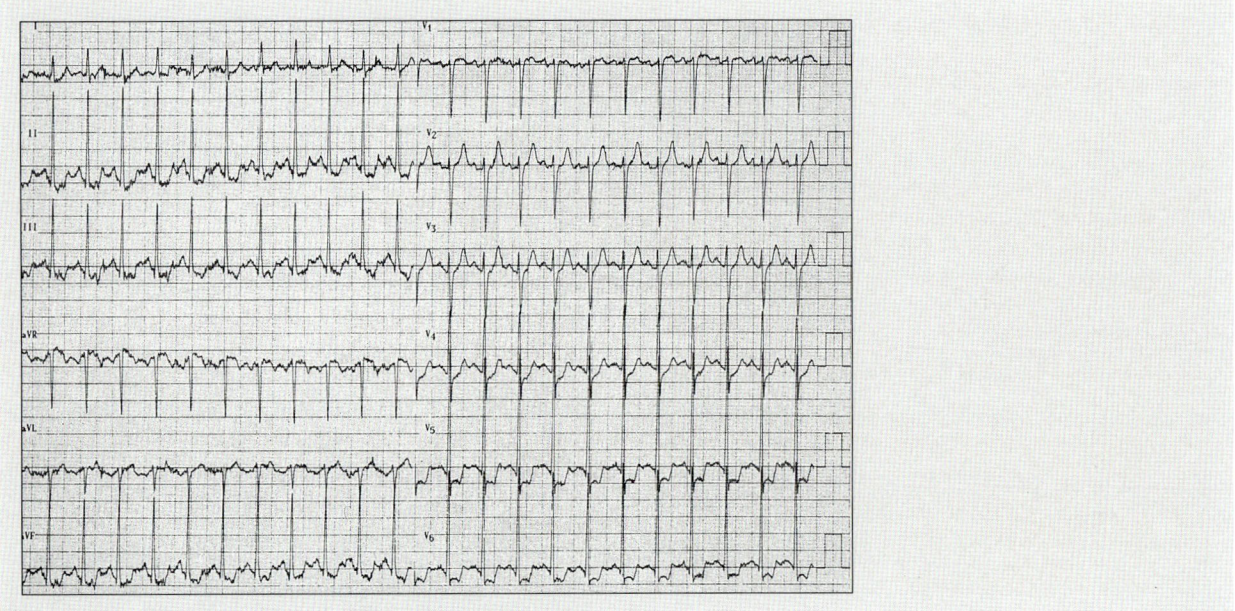

Figure 187 Exercise ECG in the same patient as in Figures 184–186 taken some weeks before the rest and exercise first-pass radionuclide angiogram. Note the significant ST segment depression in the inferior and lateral chest leads

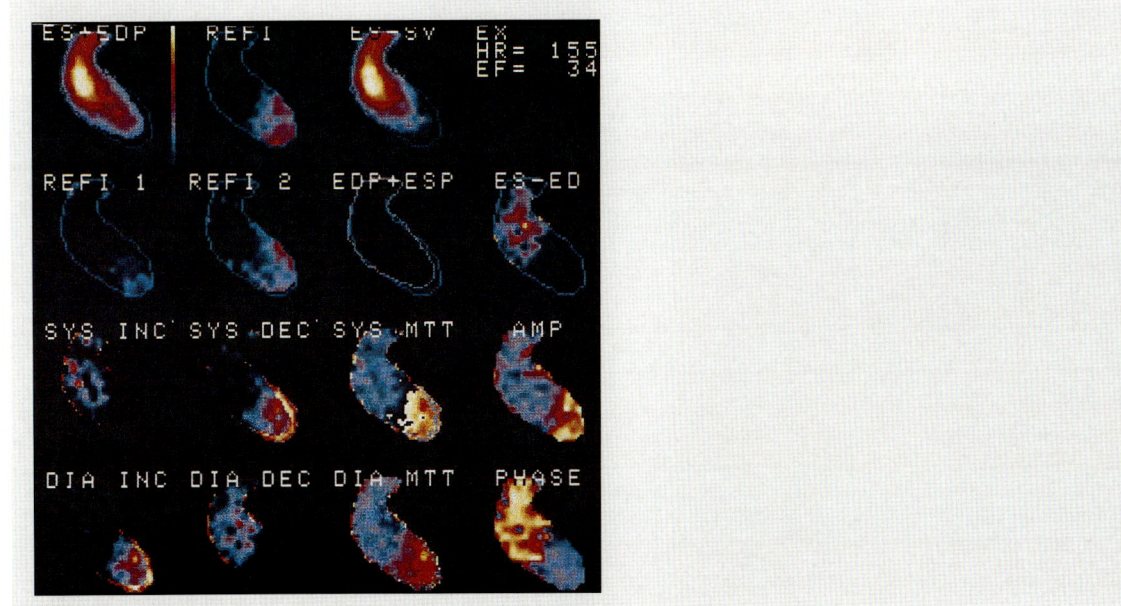

Figure 188 First-pass radionuclide angiogram after 7 min of upright bicycle exercise in the same patient as in Figures 184–187. Note that there is severe exercise-induced ischemia with the ejection fraction having fallen from 55% at rest to 34% on exercise, with a similar pattern of wall motion to that seen in Figure 184, namely global hypokinesis

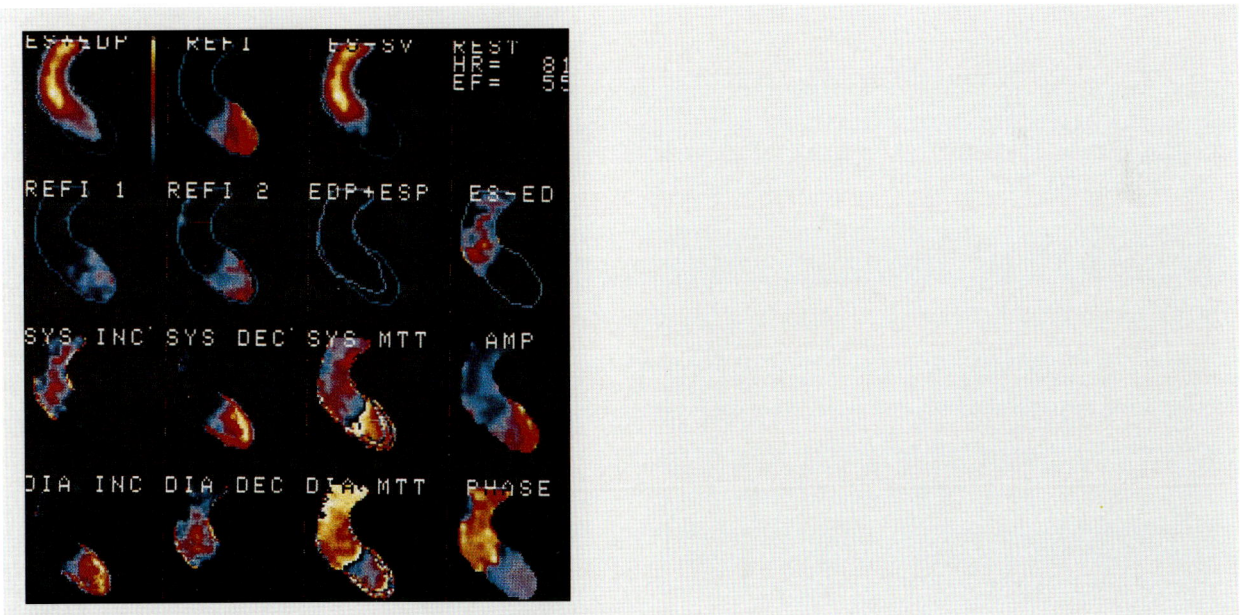

Figure 189 Resting part of a first-pass radionuclide angiogram in the same patient as in Figures 184–188 1 month after the picture shown in Figure 186 was taken. The ejection fraction is still normal at 55% with normal wall motion

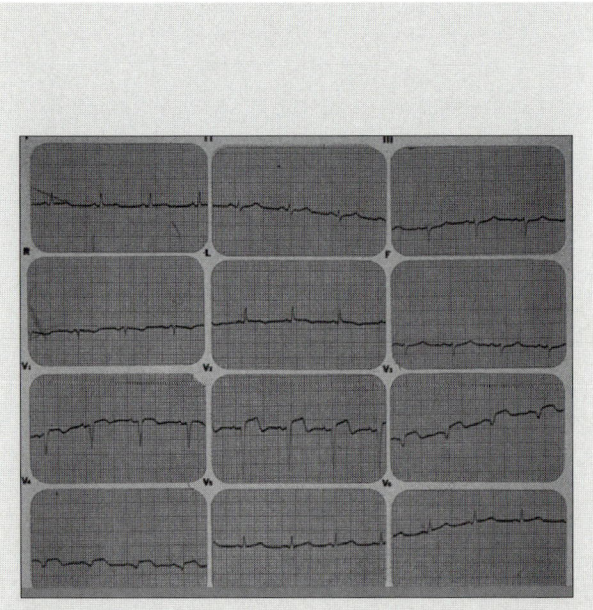

Figure 190 12-lead electrocardiogram in a patient with a completed anterior myocardial infarction with Q waves from leads VI–V4. This patient did not receive thrombolytic therapy

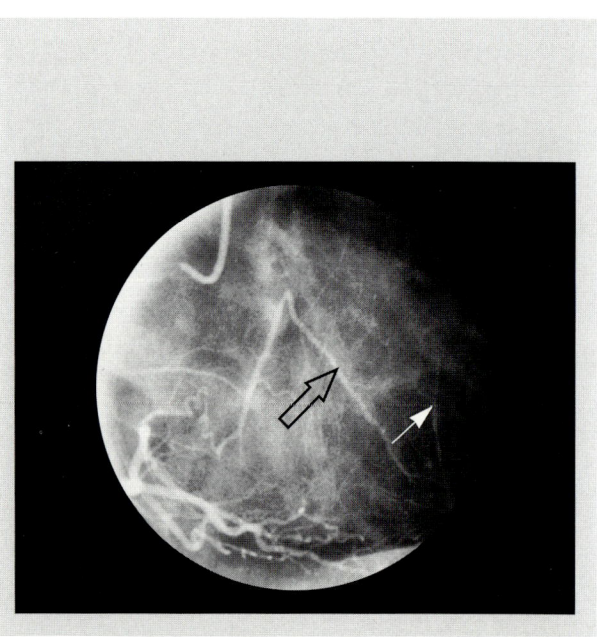

Figure 191 Late stages of a coronary angiogram in the same patient as Figure 190 in which the right coronary artery has been selectively injected. Both the circumflex (hollow arrow) and the left anterior descending (solid arrow) are seen filling retrogradely from the right coronary artery

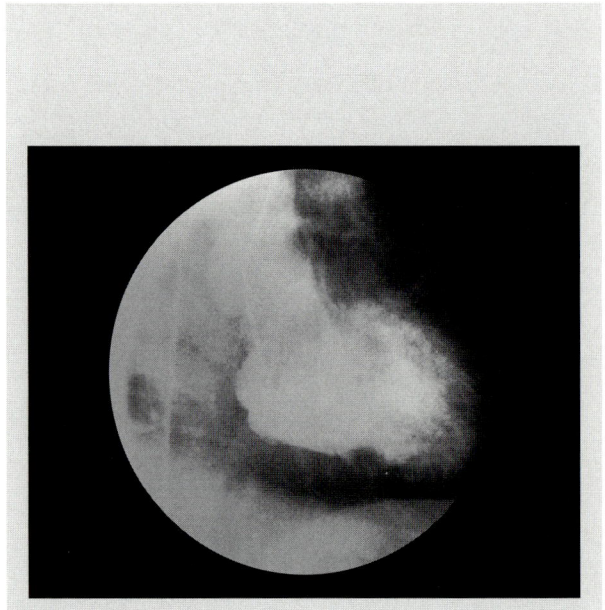

Figure 192 End-diastolic frame from the left ventricular angiogram of the same patient as in Figures 190 and 191

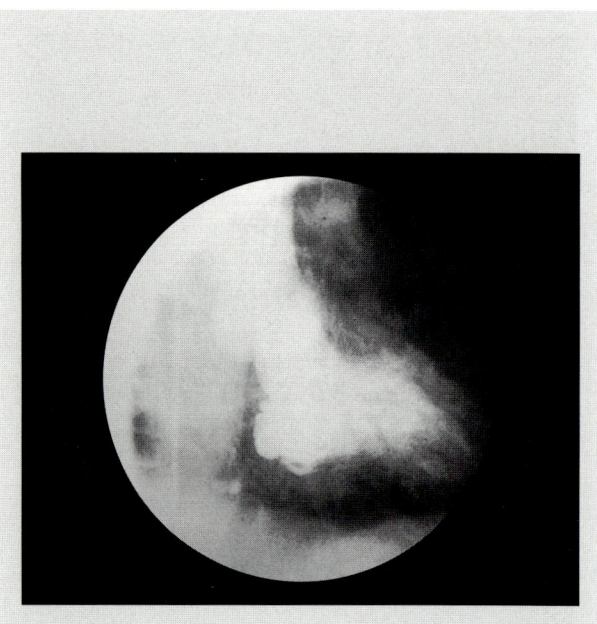

Figure 193 End-systolic frame from the left ventricular angiogram of the same patient as in Figures 190–192. It can be appreciated that there is very marked anterior wall hypokinesis, whereas there has been good inward motion of inferior wall

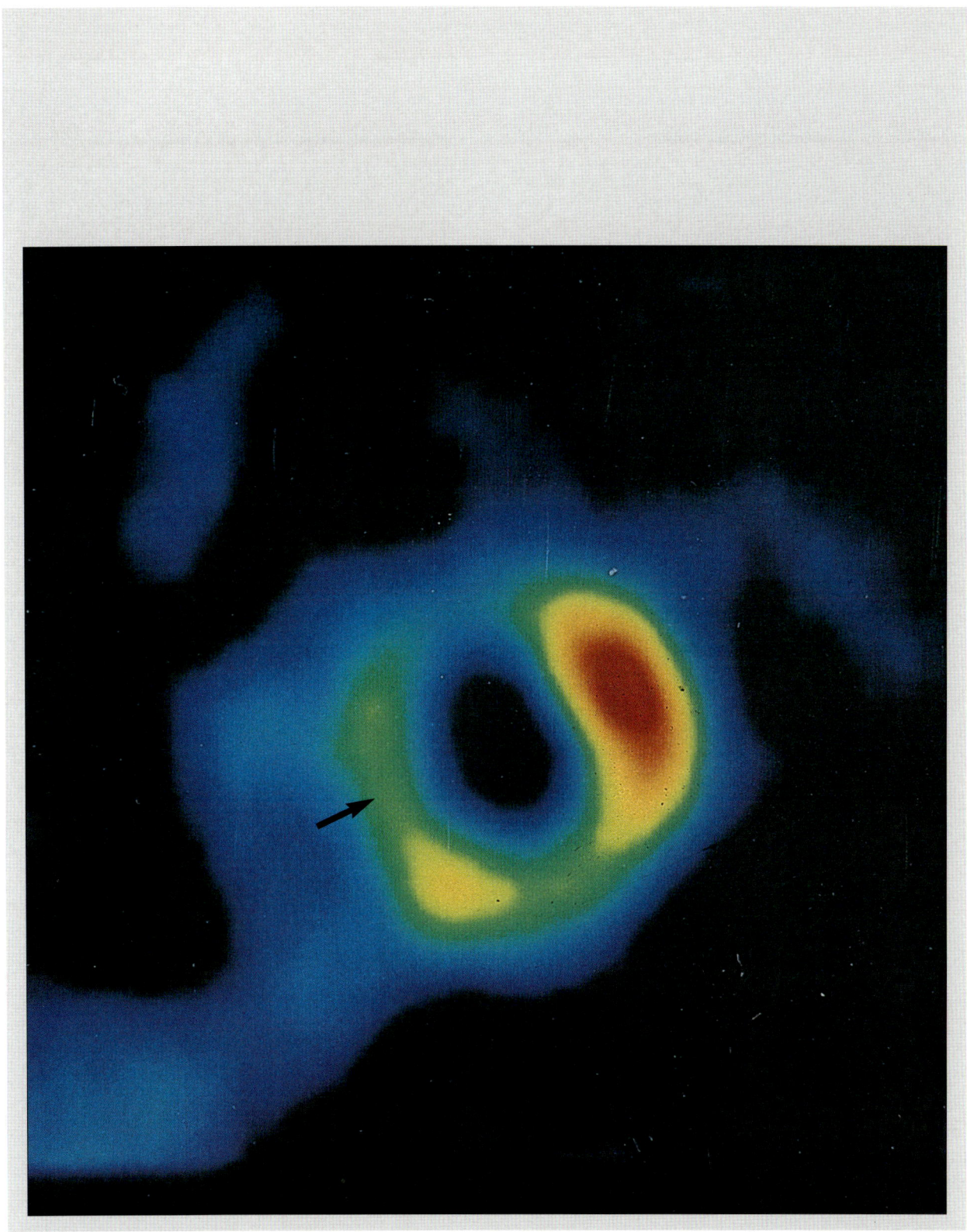

Figure 194 Tomographic cut of a thallium scan (one view from a short-axis tomogram) in the same patient as in Figures 190–193. The posterolateral wall is seen in red and yellow and the interventricular septum is seen in yellow (arrowed). Note that, in spite of the anterior Q waves and the angiographic appearances, there is still viable muscle in the septum, as manifest by the continued uptake of thallium in the arrowed region

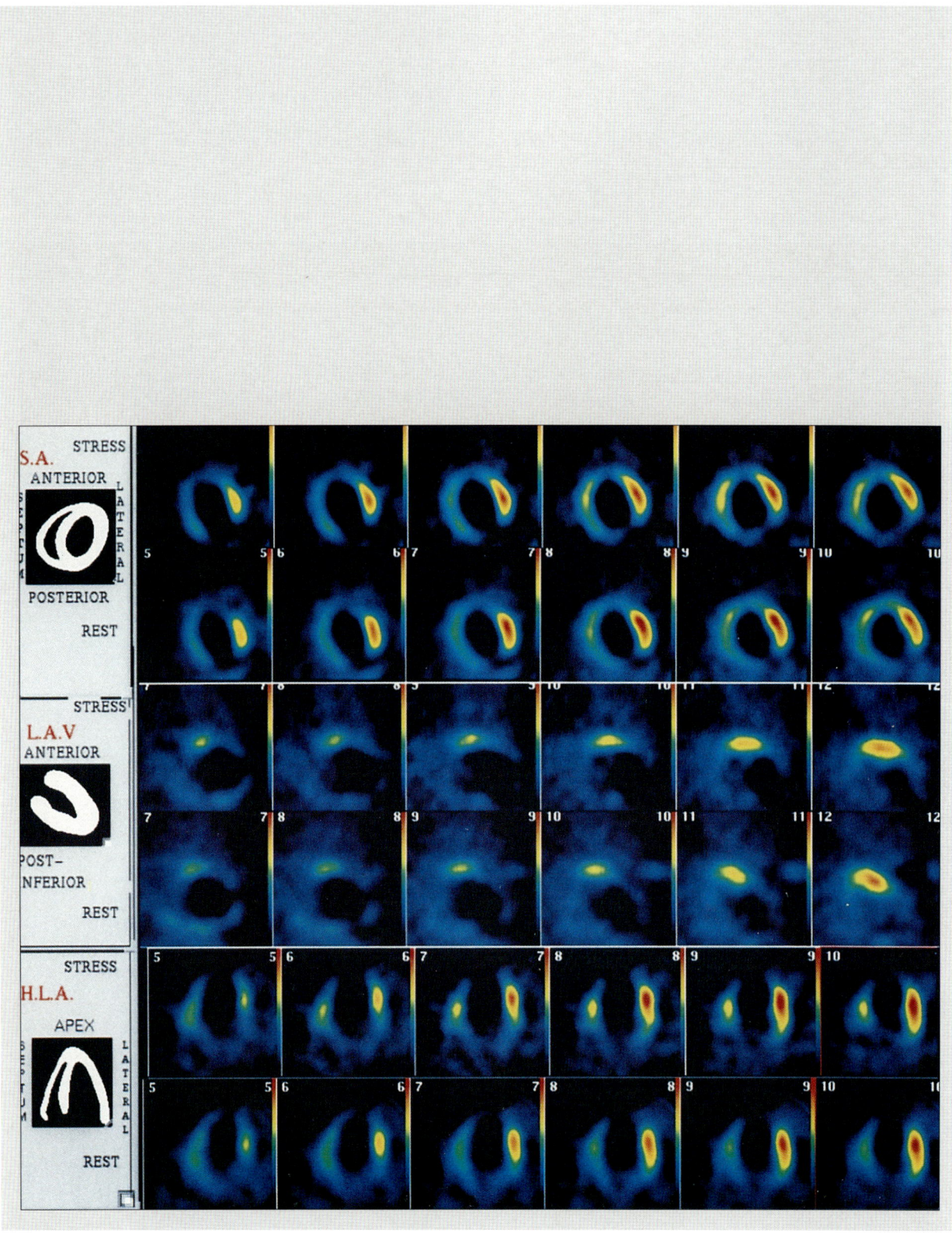

Figure 195 Thallium tomogram in three views from a patient with a very extensive anterior and inferior myocardial infarction. Scans are obtained after dipyridamole stress, and reinjection. Note the grossly reduced uptake of thallium in the septum in the short-axis views, the deficient uptake in the anterior and posteroinferior segments in the vertical long-axis tomograms, and the deficient uptake in the septum and the apical region in the horizontal long-axis tomograms. Only the posterolateral wall shows uptake of thallium and there is no difference between the two images. This indicates the absence of significant amounts of viable amounts of myocardium outside the posterolateral wall

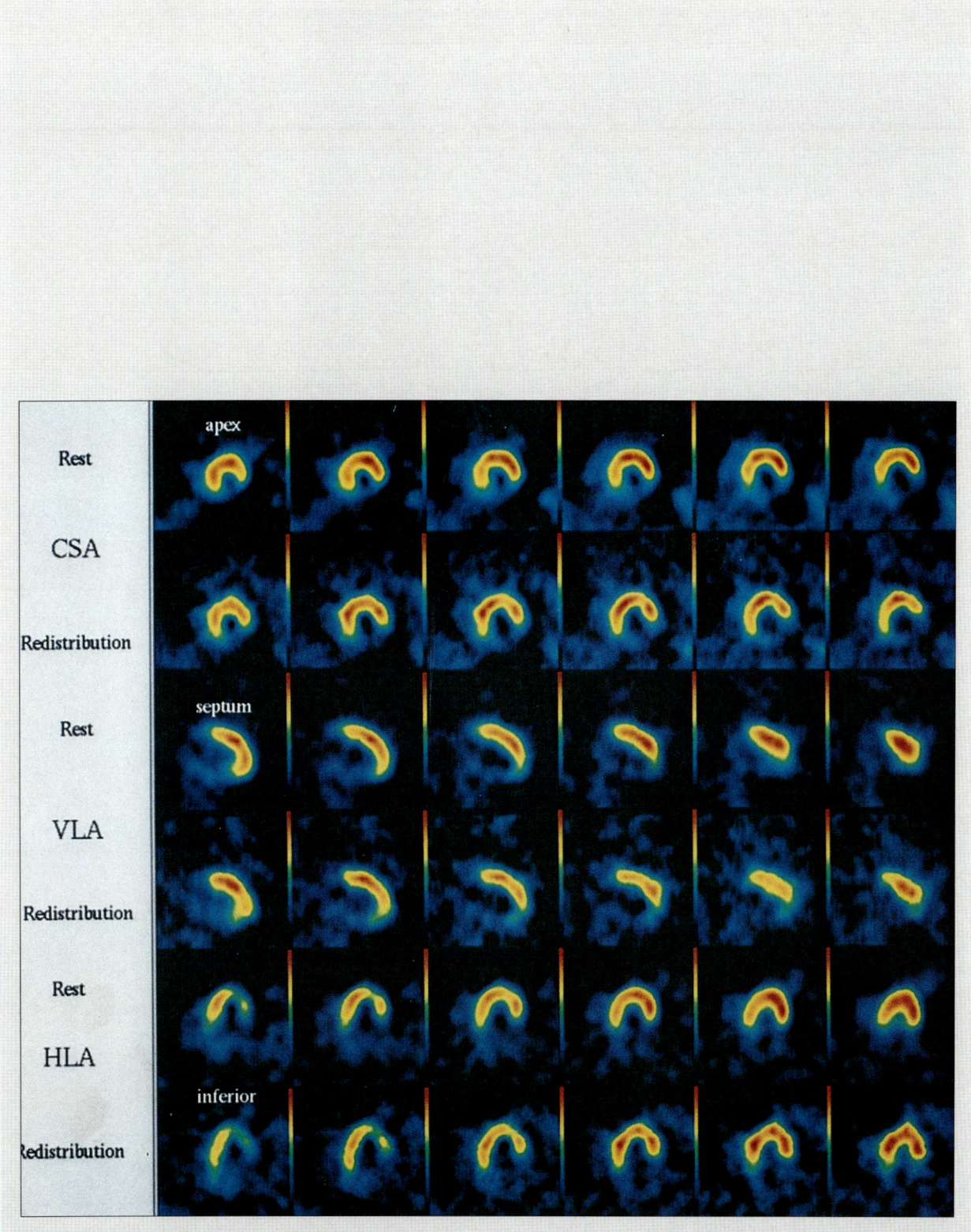

Figure 196 Rest and delayed rest (redistribution) thallium tomograms from a patient with a posteroinferior myocardial infarction. Note that on both early and late images there is deficient uptake in the posterior and inferior walls with no hint of thallium appearing in these regions. This is another example of non-viable myocardium in the territory of the posteroinferior infarction

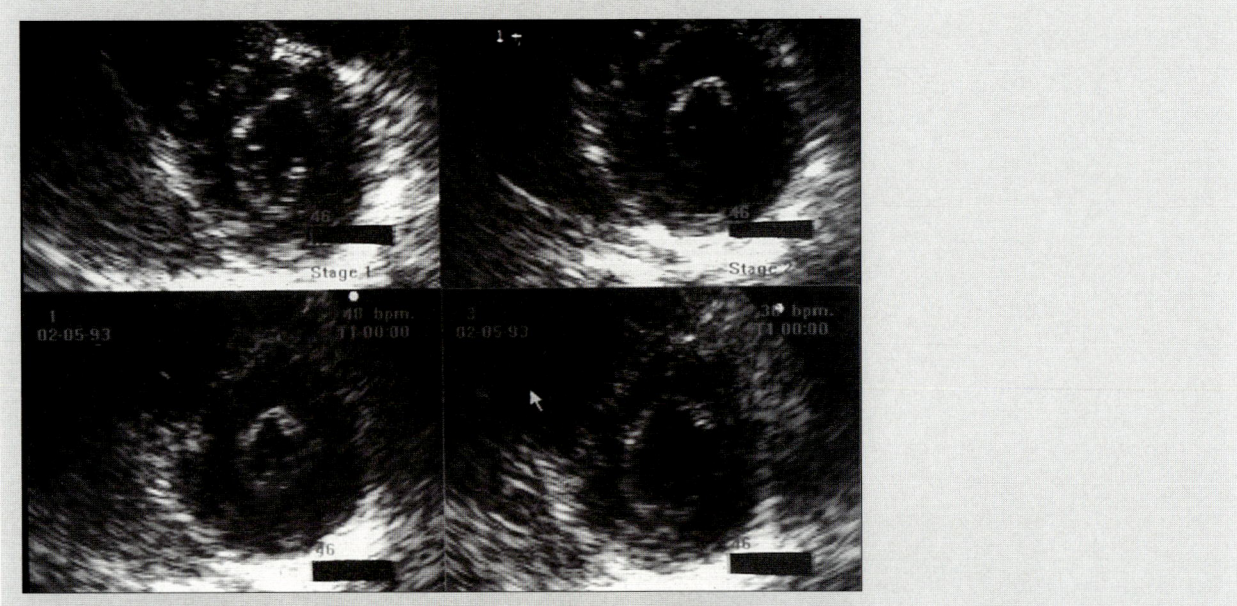

Figure 197 A normal dobutamine-stress two-dimensional echocardiogram. These are short-axis views and all are taken at end-systole. Top left (stage I): the basal condition. The thickness of the myocardium is clearly seen; note the size of the left ventricular cavity; top right (stage II): end-systolic image after low-dose dobutamine infusion. Note how the cavity size has decreased; bottom left (stage III): end-systolic frame at high-dose dobutamine infusion. Note the very small end-systolic volume indicating increased inotropic state; bottom right (stage IV): recovery. The left ventricular cavity has now returned to the same as it was in stage I

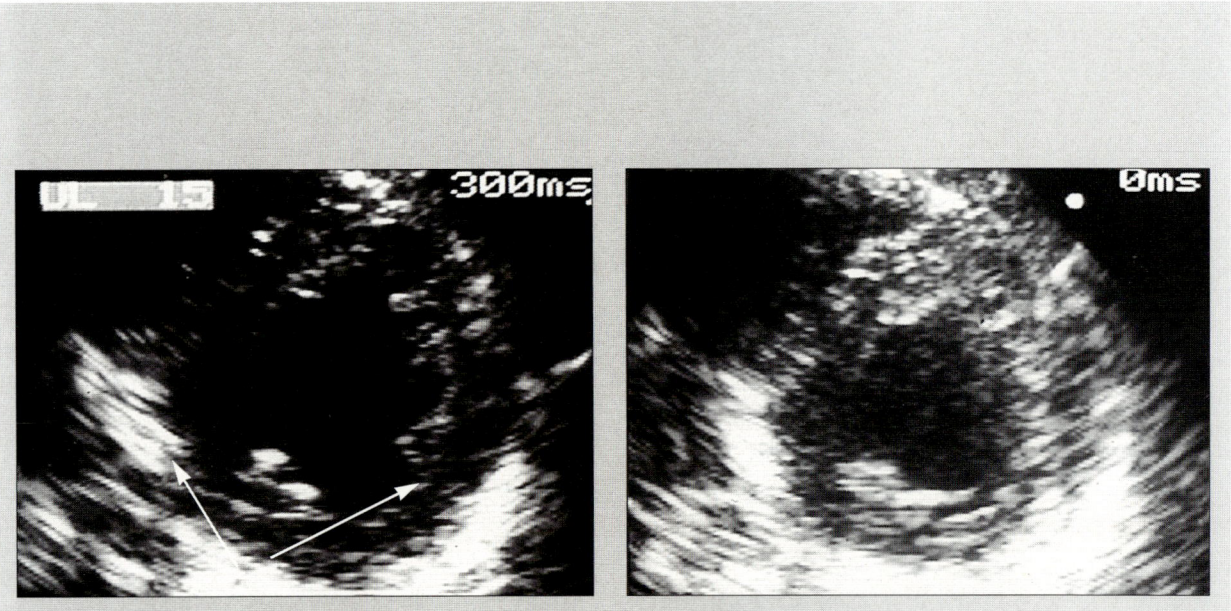

Figure 198 End-systolic short-axis two-dimensional echocardiograms in the basal state (left) and after dobutamine infusion (right). Note on the left-hand image the marked myocardial thinning of the posterior wall (arrowed). However, during dobutamine infusion there is now evidence of thickening in this region, illustrating the use of dobutamine stress echocardiography to demonstrate potentially recoverable and viable myocardium. Non-viable myocardium would not have shown such thickening during dobutamine infusion

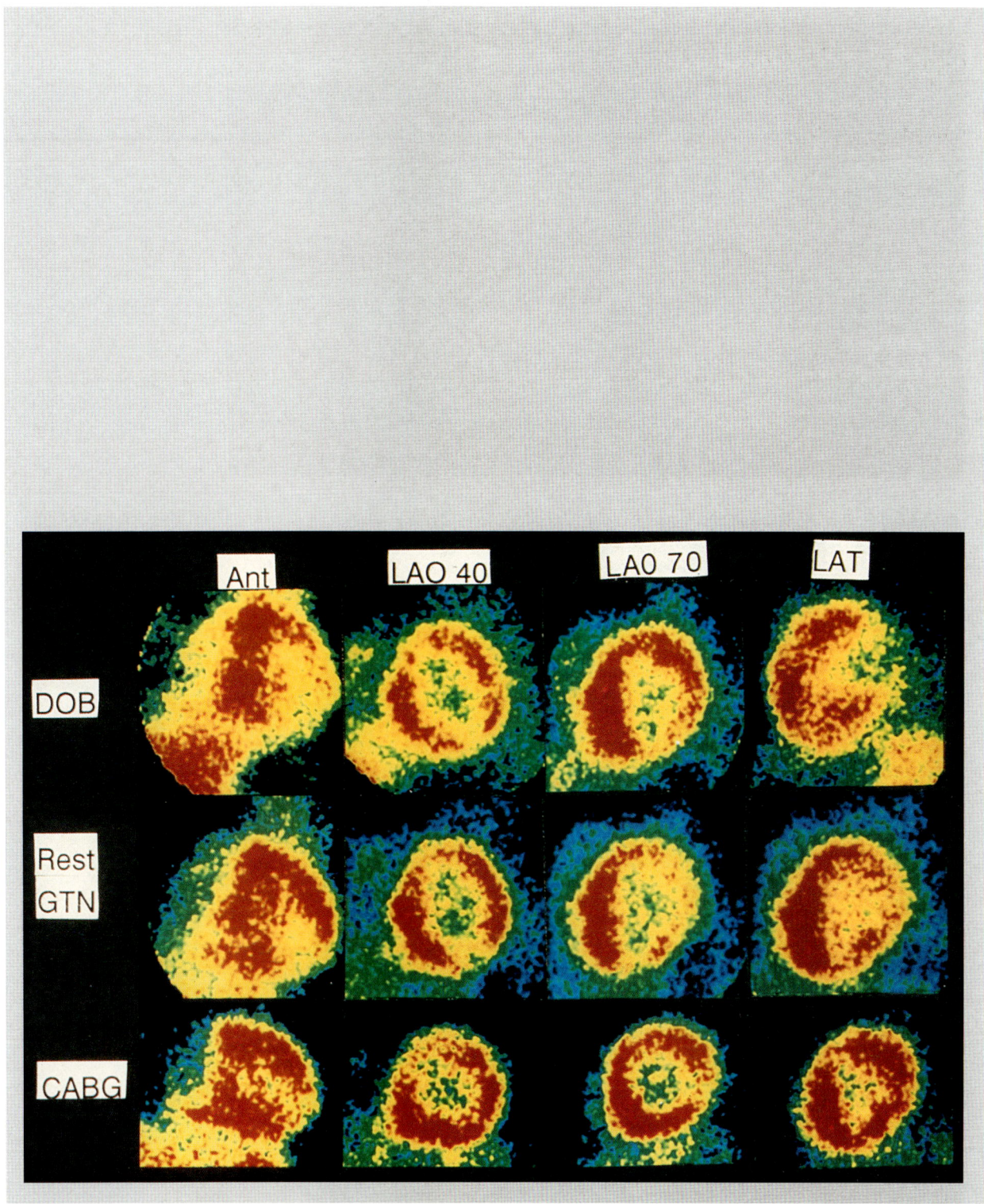

Figure 199 Planar thallium images in four projections from a patient with posterior and inferior myocardial infarction. The top four panels indicate the images after high-dose dobutamine to induce ischemia. The middle four panels show the images at rest after the administration of sublingual glyceryl trinitrate; the bottom panel shows the images after coronary artery bypass surgery. The top images show extensive defects in perfusion in the inferior wall and in the anterior wall and posterolaterally. After rest and glyceryl trinitrate, the anterior wall shows reversal of the ischemia but there are persistent defects in the inferior wall and posterior wall which suggest scar tissue. However, after coronary bypass surgery, excellent perfusion of the posterior wall is now seen and the inferior wall has also improved. High-dose dobutamine thallium scintigraphy is used to induce ischemia compared with the low-dose dobutamine echocardiography, which used to demonstrate myocardial thickening and viability

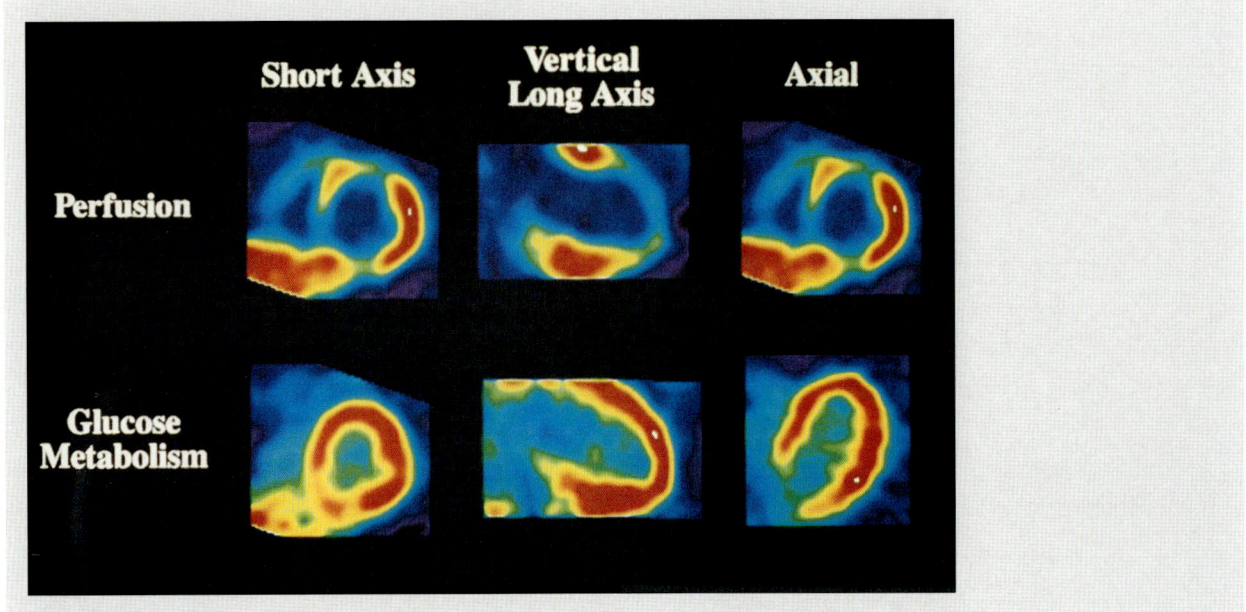

Figure 200 Positron emission tomograms showing both myocardial perfusion using ¹³N-labelled ammonia for perfusion and [¹⁸F]fluorodeoxyglucose to show glucose metabolism. These scans are from a patient with anteroseptal and posterior myocardial infarction. Good uptake is shown in yellow and red; absent uptake is blue. Note the mismatch between perfusion on the top panels and glucose metabolism in the bottom panels. This mismatch shows that, despite absent or reduced perfusion, the myocardium is still capable of metabolizing glucose and, therefore, is 'hibernating'. This sort of pattern suggests that revascularization may well lead to improvement in function of the underperfused areas

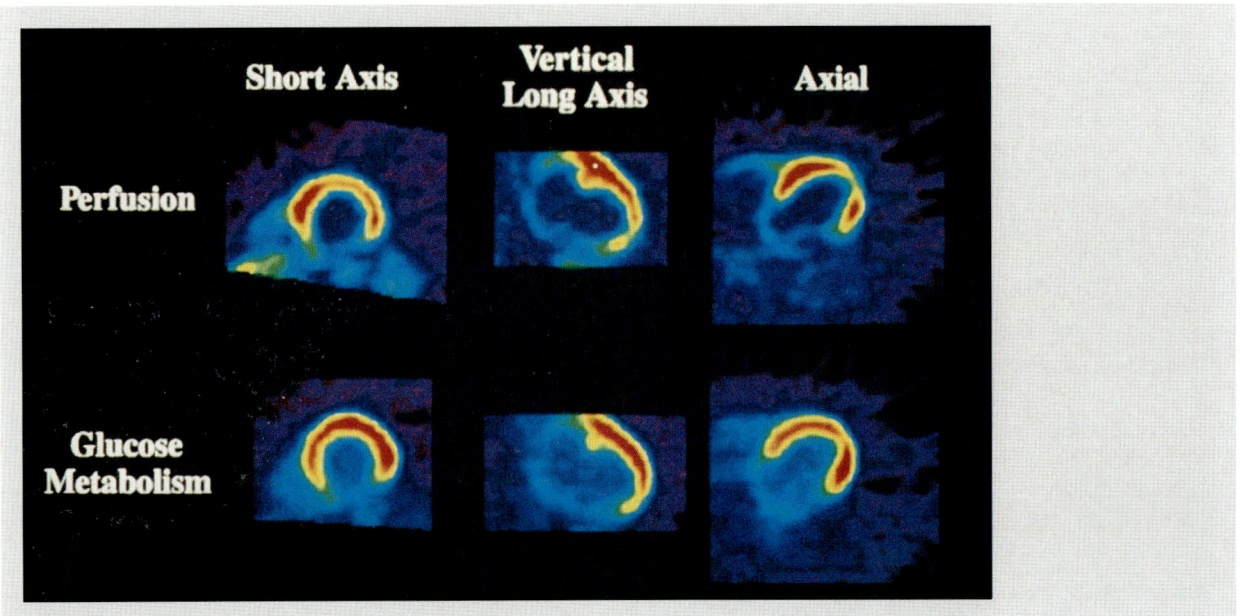

Figure 201 Same format using the same radiopharmaceuticals as in Figure 200 to show perfusion and glucose metabolism from a patient with a posterior wall myocardial infarction. Unlike Figure 200, this example shows good matching of the perfusion and glucose metabolism defects. This indicates that the muscle that has been infarcted is not viable and is scarred rather than hibernating

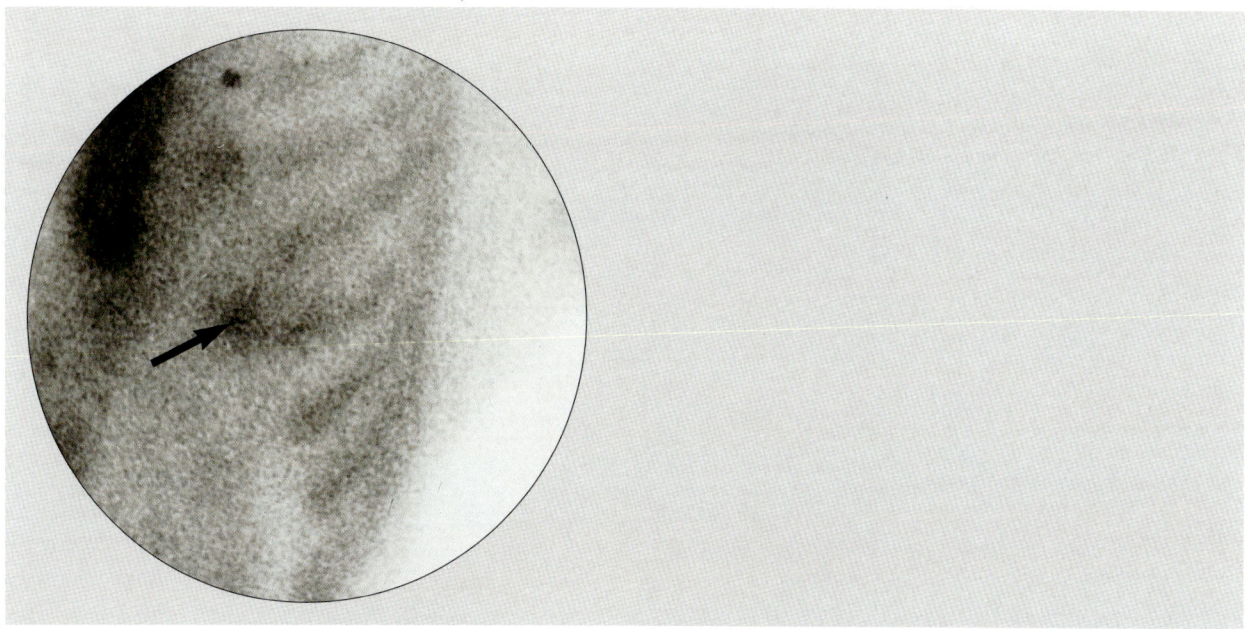

Figure 202 Anteroposterior [^{99m}Tc]pyrophosphate scan from a 23-year-old man who complained of chest pain after closed chest injury during a karate match. The patient was admitted with minor inferior wall changes on his electrocardiogram and there is a hot spot (arrowed) seen just to the left of the rib cage between the ribs and the sternum. This is an example of myocardial contusion and a subsequent coronary arteriogram was entirely normal

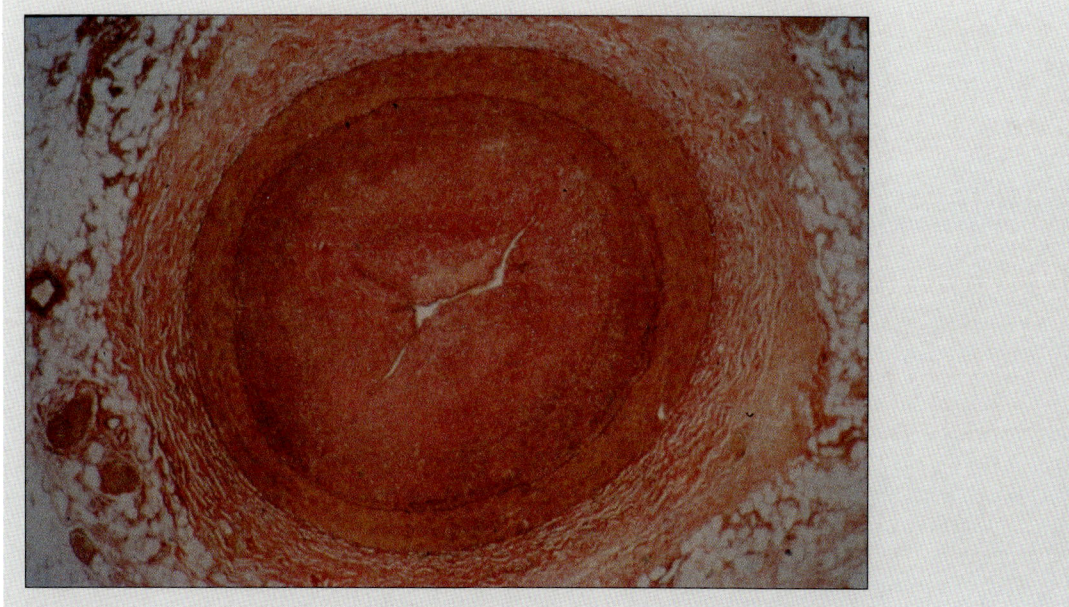

Figure 203 Histological section of an occluded coronary artery from a patient with systemic lupus erythematosis. There is no obvious arteritic inflammation but instead the lumen is filled with fresh thrombus which caused a fatal myocardial infarction. Infarction in these circumstances may be related to a hypercoagulable state in such patients who do have a tendency to produce arterial and venous thromboses even at a young age

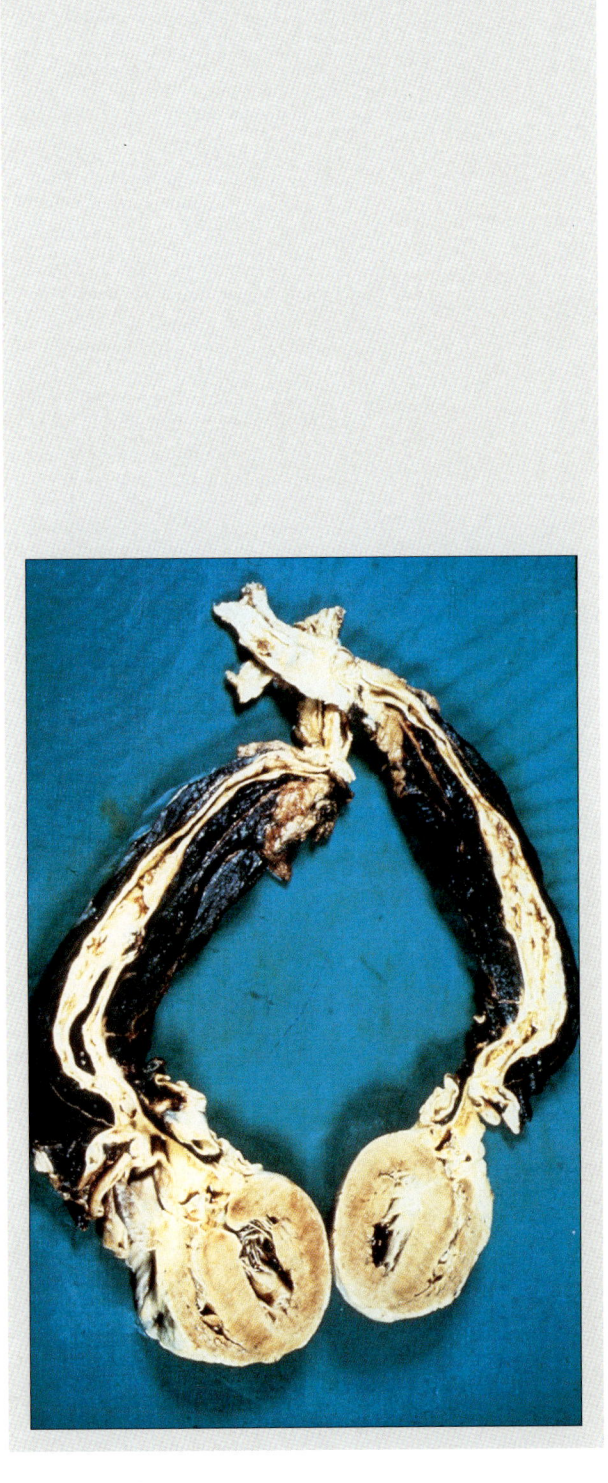

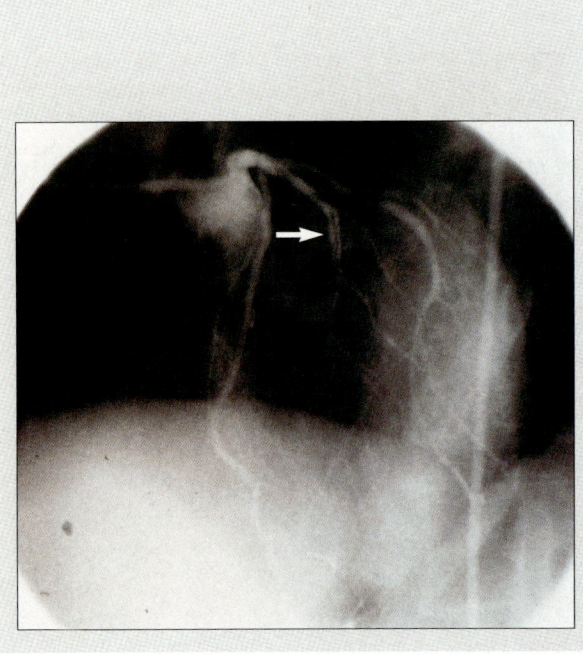

Figure 204 Postmortem heart showing massive aortic root dissection. Extensive blood clot is seen in the false lumen of the aorta. If the dissection involves the coronary ostium, then myocardial infarction may well be one of the presenting features of this syndrome

Figure 205 Left anterior oblique angiogram of the left coronary artery showing spontaneous dissection of the diagonal branch of the left anterior descending artery (arrowed). The patient presented with chest pain, lateral ECG changes and a small enzyme rise. The dissection appears as a long dark line in the artery, and a circumflex lesion is also apparent

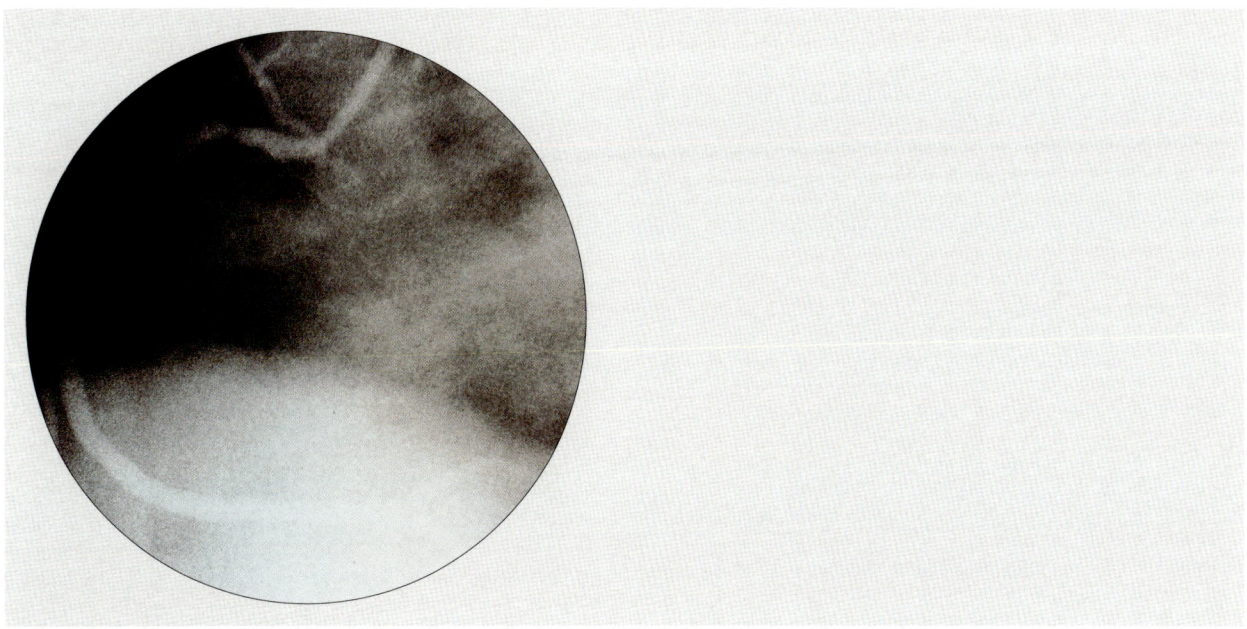

Figure 206 Iatrogenic coronary dissection. This figure shows a right coronary arteriogram from a patient with a tight proximal stenosis of the right coronary artery

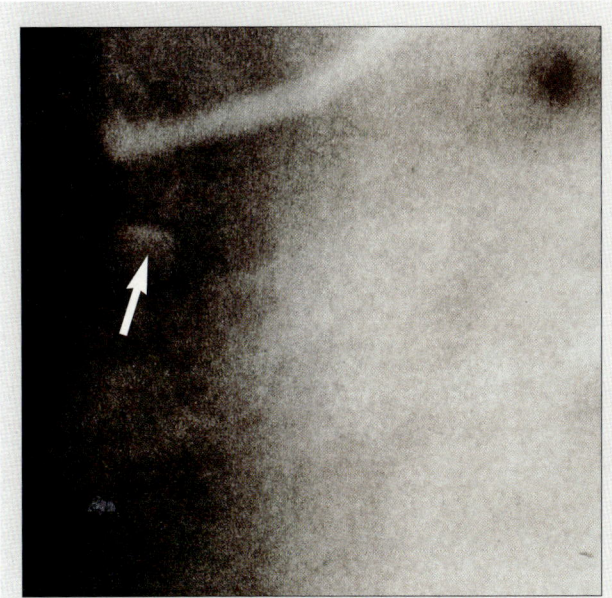
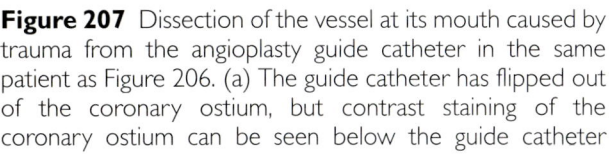
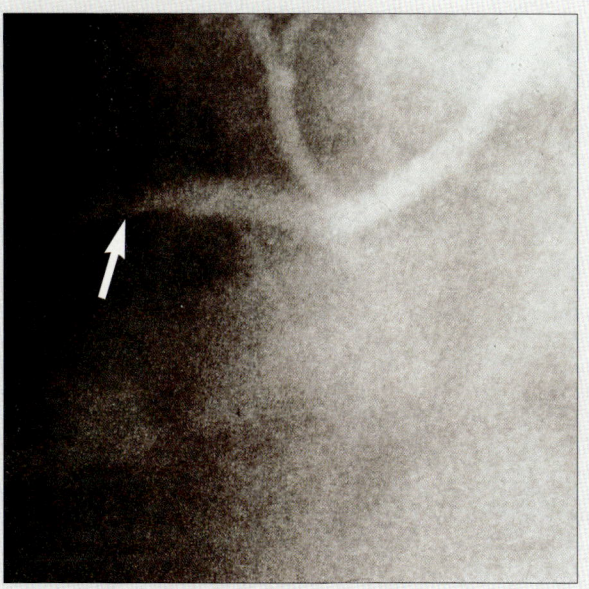

Figure 207 Dissection of the vessel at its mouth caused by trauma from the angioplasty guide catheter in the same patient as Figure 206. (a) The guide catheter has flipped out of the coronary ostium, but contrast staining of the coronary ostium can be seen below the guide catheter (arrow). (b) The coronary artery has occluded just beyond the site of the dissection (arrowed) and the patient underwent emergency coronary artery bypass surgery for a threatened substantial inferior myocardial infarction

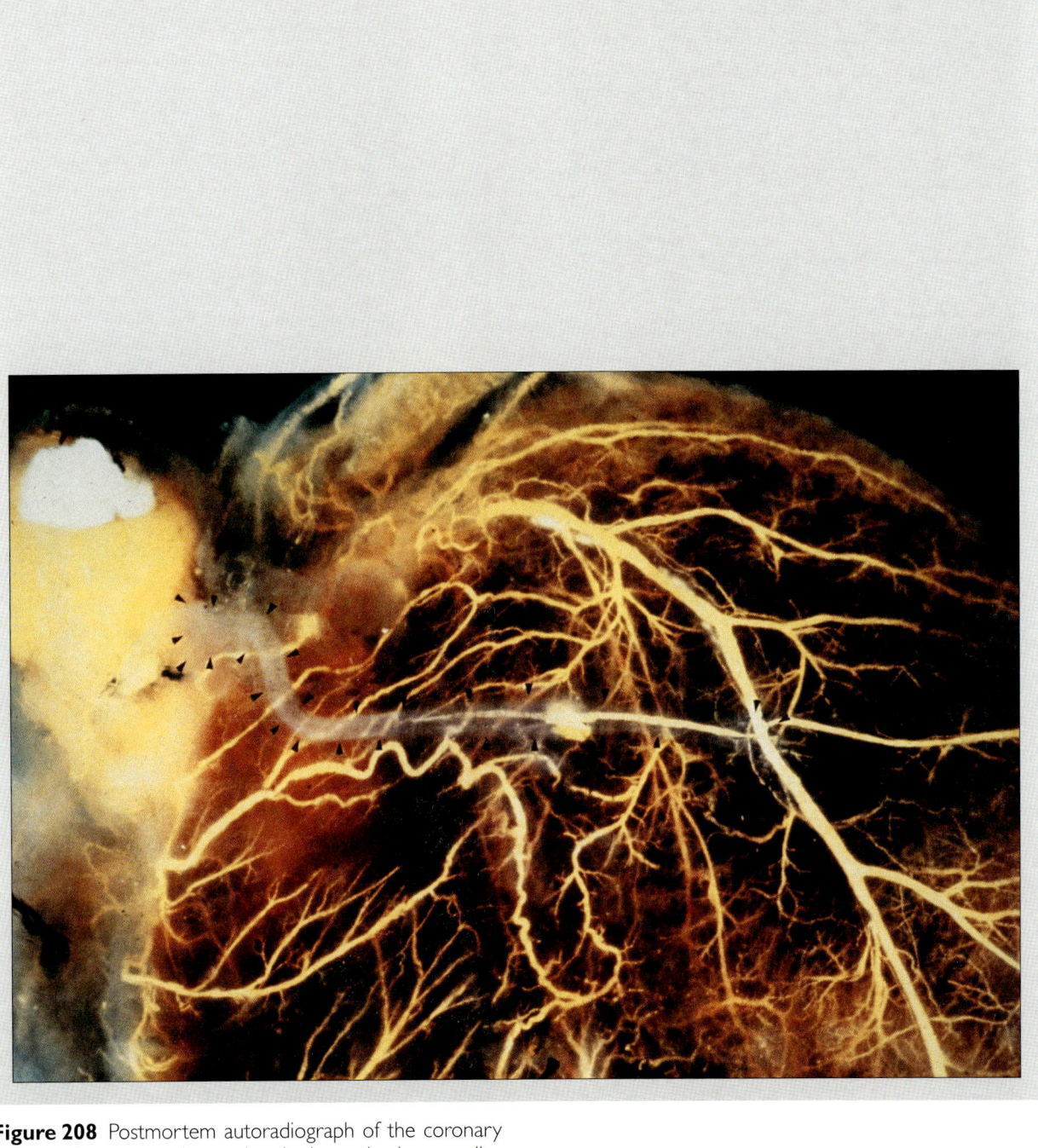

Figure 208 Postmortem autoradiograph of the coronary arteries from a patient who had received a cardiac transplantation. The small black arrows show the site of coronary occlusion and severe stenoses. Coronary artery disease in the transplanted heart is the commonest cause of mortality in cardiac transplant patients beyond 1 year

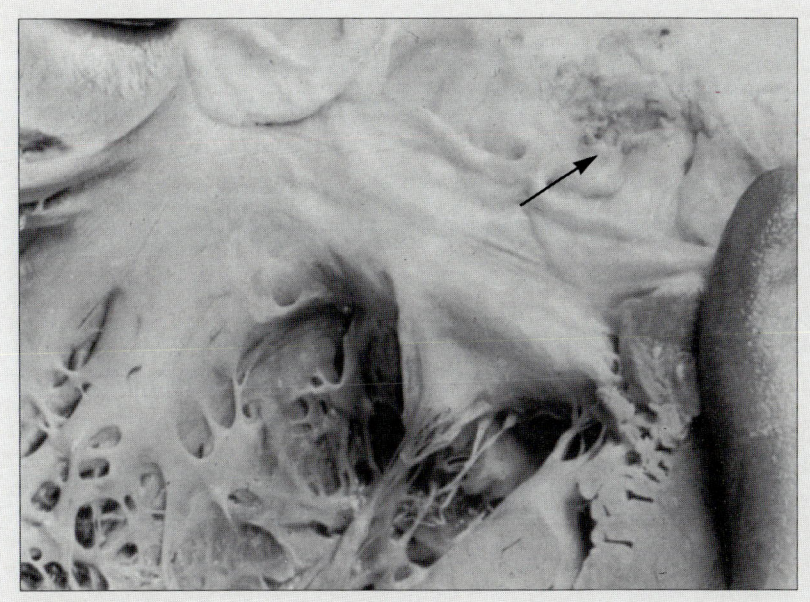

Figure 209 Postmortem heart of a patient with syphilitic aortitis showing separation of the cusps and 'tree-barking' of aorta (arrowed). Syphilitic aortitis commonly involved the coronary ostia, although it is not commonly seen nowadays

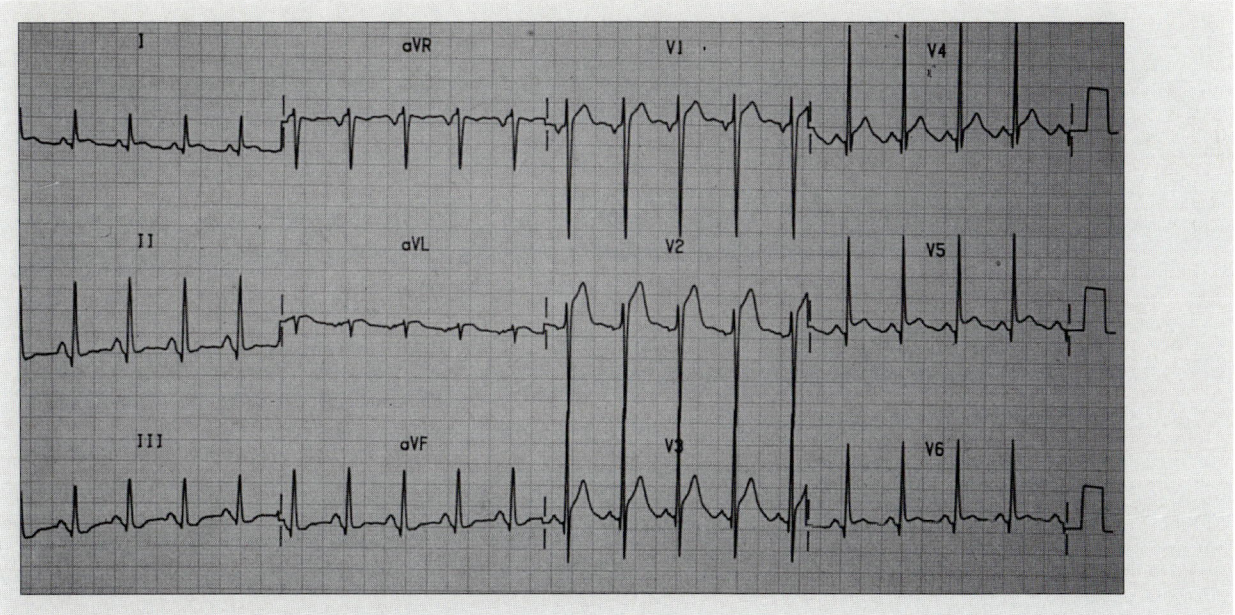

Figure 210 12-lead electrocardiogram from a patient with a pheochromocytoma receiving unopposed β-blockade. This produced a 'crisis' with chest pain and ST segment elevation in the anterior chest leads, indicating threatened acute myocardial infarction

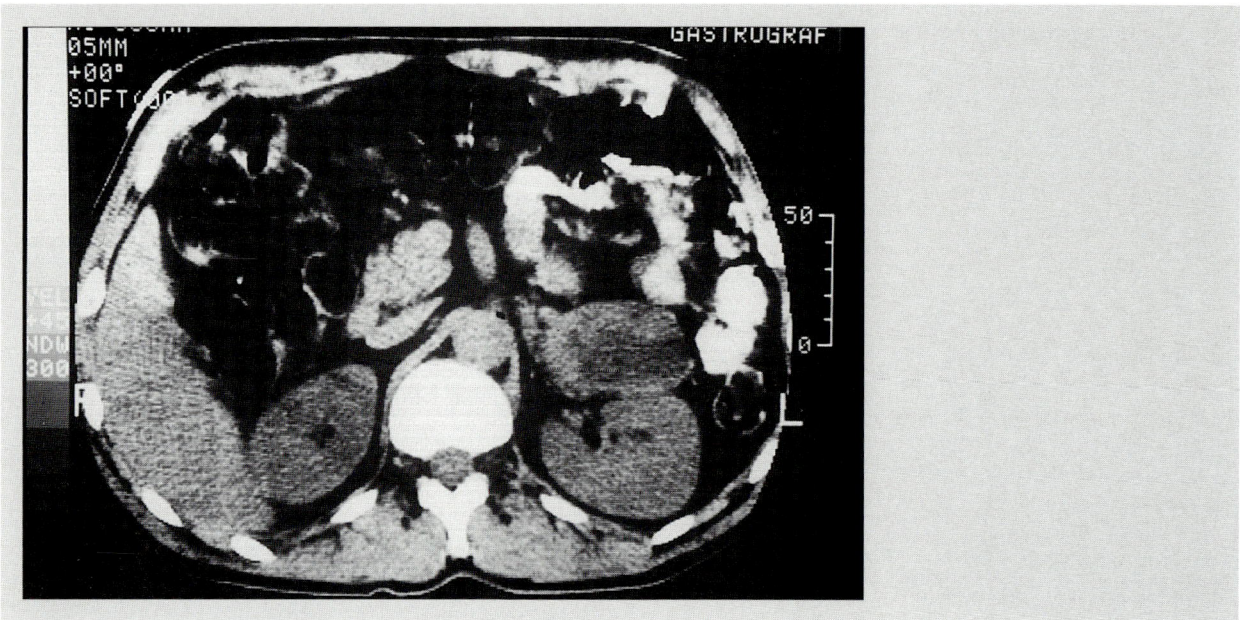

Figure 211 CT scan showing large right-sided pheochromocytoma suprarenally. There is heterogeneous contrast enhancement in the tumor

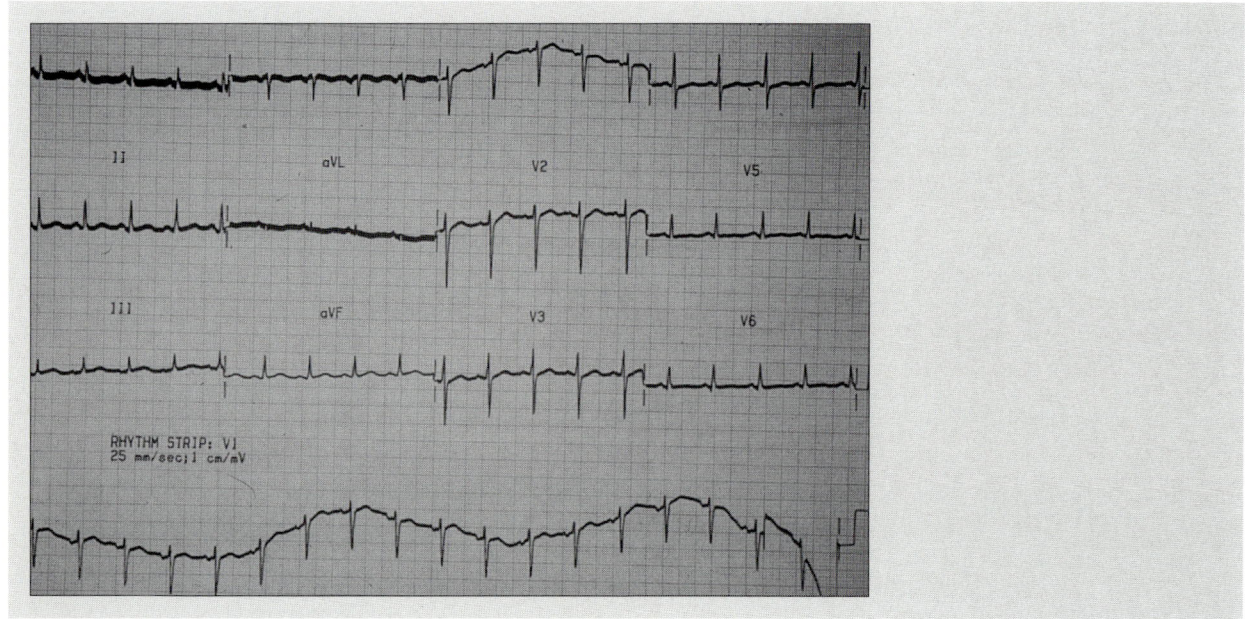

Figure 212 12-lead ECG of the same patient as in Figure 211 after resection of the tumor

Section 3   Bibliography

Benjamin-Franklin (1706–1790). 'But in this world nothing can be said to be certain, except death and taxes'. Letters to Jean Baptiste Leroy, 13 November 1789, Writings, Vol X

Epidemiology

WHO European Collaborative Group (1980). Multifactorial trial in the prevention of coronary heart disease. I. Recruitment and initial findings. *Eur. Heart J.*, **I**, 73–80

Hjerman, J. Byre, K. V., Holme, I. *et al.* (1981). Effect of diet and smoking intervention on the incidence of coronary heart disease: report from the Oslo Study Group of a randomised trial in healthy men. *Lancet*, **2**, 1303–10

Kornitzer, M., de Backer G., Dramaix, M. *et al.* (1983). Belgian Heart Disease Prevention Project: incidence and mortality results. *Lancet*, **I**, 1066–70

Goldman, L. and Cook, E. F. (1984). The decline in ischemic heart disease mortality rates: an analysis of the comparative effects of medical interventions and changes in lifestyle. *Ann. Intern. Med.*, **101**, 825–36

Lipid Research Clinics Program (1984). The Lipid Research Clinics Coronary Primary Prevention Trial Results. I. Reduction in incidence of coronary heart disease. *J. Am. Med. Assoc.*, **251**, 351–64

Shaper, A. G., Cook, D. G., Walker, M. *et al.* (1984). Prevalence of ischaemic heart disease in middle aged British men. *Br. Heart J.*, **51**, 606–11

Shaper, A. G., Pocock, S. J., Walker, M. *et al.* (1985). Risk factors for ischaemic heart disease; the prospective phase of the British Regional Heart Study. *J. Epidemiol. Community Health,* **39**, 197–209

Sytkowski, P. A., Kannel, W. B. and D'agostino, R. B. (1990). Changes in risk factors and the decline in mortality from cardiovascular disease: the Framingham Heart Study. *N. Engl. J. Med.*, **322**, 1635–41

Shaper, A. G. and Wannamethee, G. (1991). Physical activity and ischaemic heart disease in middle aged British men. *Br. Heart J.*, **66**, 384–94

Pathophysiology and plaque rupture

Paul, O. (1974). Myocardial infarction and sudden death. In Braunwald, E. (ed.) *The Myocardium; Failure and Infarction,* pp. 273–82. (New York: HP Publishing)

Lovegrove, T. and Thompson, P. (1978). The role of acute myocardial infarction in sudden cardiac death. A statistician's nightmare (editorial). *Am. Heart J.*, **96**, 711–13

Wissler, R. W. (1984). Principles of the pathogenesis of atherosclerosis in heart disease. In Braunwald, E. (ed.) *A Textbook of Cardiovascular Medicine,* 2nd edn., pp. 1183–204. (Chicago: W B Saunders)

Davies, M. J. and Thomas, A. C. (1985). Plaque fissuring – the cause of acute myocardial infarction, sudden ischaemic death and crescendo angina. *Br. Heart J.*, **53**, 363–73

Muller, J. E., Stone, P. E., Turi, Z. G. *et al.* and MILIS Study Group (1985). Circadian variation in the frequency of onset of acute myocardial infarction. *N. Engl. J. Med.*, **313**, 1315–22

Barger, A.C. and Beeuwkes, R. III. (1990). Rupture of coronary vasa vasorum as a trigger of acute myocardial infarction. *Am. J. Cardiol.*, **66**, 41–3G

Constantinides, P. (1990). Cause of thrombosis in human atherosclerotic arteries. *Am. J. Cardiol.*, **66**, 37–40G

Gertz, S.D., Kragel, A.H., Kalan, J.M. *et al.* (1990). Comparison of coronary and myocardial morphologic findings in patients with and without thrombolytic therapy during fatal acute myocardial infarction. *Am. J. Cardiol.*, **66**, 904–9

Stone, P.H. (1990). Triggers of transient myocardial ischemia: circadian variation and relation to plaque rupture and coronary thrombosis in stable coronary artery disease. *Am. J. Cardiol.*, **66**, 32–6G

Tofler, G.H., Stone, P.H., Maclure, M. *et al.* (1990). Analysis of possible triggers of acute myocardial infarction (the MILIS study). *Am. J. Cardiol.*, **66**, 22–7

Willich, S.N. (1990). Epidemiologic studies demonstrating increased morning incidence of sudden death. *Am. J. Cardiol.*, **66**, 15–17G

Primary ventricular fibrillation

DuBois, C., Smeets, J.P., DeMoulin, J.C. *et al.* (1986). Incidence, clinical significance and prognosis of ventricular fibrillation in early phase of myocardial infarction. *Eur. Heart J.*, **7**, 945–51

Behar, S., Goldbourt, U., Reicher-Reiss, H. *et al.* and SPRINT investigators (1990). Prognosis of acute myocardial infarction complicated by primary ventricular fibrillation. *Am. J. Cardiol.*, **66**, 1208–11

Jensen, G.V.H., Torp-Pedersen, C., Kober, L. *et al.* (1990). Prognosis of late versus early ventricular fibrillation in acute myocardial infarction. *Am. J. Cardiol.*, **66**, 10–15

Reciprocal ECG change

Gibson, R.S., Crampton, R.S., Watson, D.D. *et al.* (1982). Precordial ST segment depression during acute inferior myocardial infarction: clinical, scintigraphic and angiographic correlations. *Circulation*, **66**, 732–41

Strasberg, B., Pinchas, A., Barbash, G.I. *et al.* (1990). Importance of reciprocal ST segment depression in leads V5 and V6 as an indicator of disease of the left anterior descending coronary artery in acute inferior wall myocardial infarction. *Br. Heart J.*, **63**, 339–41

Thrombolysis

Simoons, M.L., van den Brand, M., de Zwaan, C. *et al.* (1985). Improved survival after early thrombolysis in acute myocardial infarction: a randomised trial by the Interuniversity Cardiology Institute in The Netherlands. *Lancet*, **2**, 578–81

The TIMI study group (1985). The thrombolysis in myocardial infarction (TIMI) trial. Phase I findings. *N. Engl. J. Med.*, **312**, 932–6

DeWood, M.A., Stifter, W.F., Simpson, C.S. *et al.* (1986). Coronary arteriographic findings soon after non Q wave myocardial infarction. *N. Engl. J. Med.*, **315**, 417–23

Gruppo Italiano per lo Studio della Streptochinasi nell Infarto Miocardico (GISSI) (1986). Effectiveness of intravenous thrombolytic treatment in acute myocardial infarction. *Lancet*, **1**, 397–402

Topol, E.J., Califf, R.M., George, G.S. *et al.* and TAMI study group (1987). A randomized trial of immediate versus delayed elective angioplasty after intravenous tissue plasminogen activator in acute myocardial infarction. *N. Engl. J. Med.*, **317**, 581–8

ISIS-2 (Second International Study of Infarct Survival) Collaborative Group (1988). Randomised trial of intravenous streptokinase, oral aspirin, both or neither among 17187 cases of suspected acute myocardial infarction. *Lancet*, **2**, 349–60

Wilcox, R.G., van der Lippe, G., Olson, C.G. *et al.* (1988). Trial of tissue plasminogen activator for mortality reduction in acute myocardial infarction. Anglo-Scandinavian Study of Early Thrombolysis (ASSET). *Lancet*, **2**, 525–30

The TIMI Study Group (1989). Comparison of invasive and conservative strategies after treatment with intravenous tissue plasminogen activator in acute myocardial infarction: results of the thrombolysis in Myocardial Infarction (TIMI) Phase II Trial. *N. Engl. J. Med.*, **320**, 618–27

AIMS Trial Study Group (1990). Long-term effects of intravenous anistreplase in acute myocardial infarction: final report of the AIMS study. *Lancet*, **335**, 427–31

Gruppo Italiano per lo Studio della Sopravivenza nell Infarto Miocardico GISSI-2 (1990). A factorial randomised trial of alteplase versus streptokinase and heparin vs no heparin among 12490 patients with acute myocardial infarction. *Lancet,* **336**, 65–71

Hsia, J., Hamilton, W.P., Kleiman, N. *et al.* (1990). A comparison between heparin and low dose aspirin as adjunctive therapy with tissue plasminogen activator for acute myocardial infarction. *N. Engl. J. Med.,* **223**, 1433–7

ISIS-3 (Third International Study of Infarct Survival) Collaborative Group (1992). ISIS-3: A randomised comparison of streptokinase vs tissue plasminogen activator vs anistreplase and of aspirin plus heparin vs aspirin alone among 41299 cases of suspected acute myocardial infarction. *Lancet,* **339**, 753–70

Krumholz, H.M., Pasternak, R.C., Weinstein, M.L. *et al.* (1992). Cost-effectiveness of thrombolytic therapy with streptokinase in elderly patients with suspected acute myocardial infarction. *N. Engl. J. Med.,* **327**, 7–13

Kleiman, N.S., Ohman, E.M., Califf, R.M. *et al.* (1993). Profound inhibition of platelet aggregation with monoclonal antibody of 7E3 Fab after thrombolytic therapy. Results of the thrombolysis and angioplasty in myocardial infarction (TAMI) 8 study. *J. Am. Coll. Cardiol.,* **22**, 381–9

Linderer, T., Schröder, R., Arnoz, R. *et al.* (1993). Pre-hospital thrombolysis; beneficial effect of very early treatment on infarct size and left ventricular function. *J. Am. Coll. Cardiol.,* **22**, 1304–10

Veen, G., Meyer, A., Verheugt, F.W.A. *et al.* (1993). Culprit lesion morphology and stenosis severity in the prediction of reocclusion after coronary thrombolysis: angiographic results of the APRICOT study. *J. Am. Coll. Cardiol.,* **22**, 1755–62

Primary angioplasty

O'Keefe, J.H., Rutherford, B.D., McConohay, D.A. *et al.* (1989). Early and late results of coronary angioplasty without antecedent thrombolytic therapy for acute myocardial infarction. *Am. J. Cardiol.,* **64**, 1221–30

Grines, C.L., Browne, K.F., Marco, J. *et al.* (1993). For the Primary Angioplasty in Myocardial Infarction (PAMI) study group. A comparison of immediate angioplasty with thrombolytic therapy for acute myocardial infarction. *N. Engl. J. Med.,* **328**, 673–9

Himbert, D., Juliard, J.-M., Steg, G. *et al.* (1993). Primary coronary angioplasty for acute myocardial infarction with contra-indication to thrombolysis. *Am. J. Cardiol.,* **71**, 377–81

Santiago, P., Vacek, J.L., Rosamond, T.L. *et al.* (1993). Comparison of results of coronary angioplasty during acute myocardial infarction with and without previous coronary bypass surgery. *Am. J. Cardiol.,* **72**, 1348–51

Zijlstra, F., de Boer, M.J., Hoorntje, J.C.A. *et al.* (1993). A comparison of immediate coronary angioplasty with intravenous streptokinase in acute myocardial infarction. *N. Engl. J. Med.,* **328**, 680–4

β-Blockade

Yusuf, S., Peto, R., Lewis, J. *et al.* (1985). Beta blockade during and after myocardial infarction: an overview of the randomized trials. *Prog. Cardiovasc. Dis.,* **27**, 335–71

Byington, R.P., Worthy, J., Craven, T. *et al.* (1990). Propranolol-induced lipid changes and their prognostic significance after a myocardial infarction: the Beta Blocker Heart Attack experience. *Am. J. Cardiol.,* **65**, 1287–91

Prognosis after infarction

Theroux, P., Waters, D.D., Halphen, C. *et al.* (1979). Prognostic value of exercise testing soon after myocardial infarction. *N. Engl. J. Med.,* **301**, 341–5

Starling, M.R., Crawford, M.H., Kennedy, G.T. *et al.* (1980). Exercise testing early after myocardial infarction: predictive value for subsequent unstable angina and death. *Am. J. Cardiol.,* **46**, 909–14

Moss, A.J. (1982). Prognosis after myocardial infarction. *Am. J. Cardiol.,* **52**, 667–9

Bratt, S.H., de Zwaan, C., Brugada, P. *et al.* (1983). Values of left ventricular ejection fraction in extensive anterior infarction to predict development of ventricular tachycardia. *Am. J. Cardiol.,* **52**, 686–91

Gibson, R.S., Watson, D.D., Craddock, G.B. *et al.* (1983). Prediction of cardiac events after uncomplicated myocardial infarction: a prospective study comparing pre-discharge exercise thallium-201 scintigraphy and coronary angiography. *Circulation,* **68**, 321–36

Bigger, J.T., Fleiss, J.L., Kleiger, R. *et al.* (1984). The Multicenter Postinfarction Research Group; the relationships among ventricular arrhythmias, left ventricular dysfunction and mortality in the two years after myocardial infarction. *Circulation,* **69**, 250–8

Gottlieb, S., Gottlieb, S., Achuff, S. *et al.* (1988). Silent ischemia on Holter monitoring predicts mortality in high risk post infarction patients. *J. Am. Med. Assoc.,* **259**, 1030–41

Goldberg, R. J., Gore, J. M., Gurwitz, J. H. *et al.* (1989). The impact of age on the incidence and prognosis of initial acute myocardial infarction: the Worcester Heart Attack Study. *Am. Heart J.*, **117**, 543–9

Gunnar, R. M., Passamani, E. R., Bourdillon, P. D. *et al.* (1990). Guidelines for the early management of patients with acute myocardial infarction: a report of the American College of Cardiology/American Heart Association Task Force on Assessment of Diagnostic and Therapeutic Cardiovascular Procedures (subcommittee to develop guidelines for the early management of patients with acute myocardial infarction). *J. Am. Coll. Cardiol.*, **16**, 249–92

Smith, P., Arnesen, W. and Holme, I. (1990). The effect of warfarin on mortality and reinfarction after myocardial infarction. *N. Engl. J. Med.*, **323**, 147–52

Mueller, H. S., Cohen, L. S., Braunwald, E. *et al.* (1992). Predictors of early morbidity and mortality after thrombolytic therapy of acute myocardial infarction. Analysis of patient subgroups in the thrombolysis in myocardial infarction (TIMI) trial, phase II. *Circulation*, **85**, 1254–64

Petretta, M., Bonaduce, D., Bianchi, V. *et al.* (1992). Characterization and prognostic significance of silent myocardial ischemia on predischarge electrocardiographic monitoring in unselected patients with myocardial infarction. *Am. J. Cardiol.*, **69**, 579–83

Galvani, M., Ottani, F., Ferrini, D. *et al.* (1993). Patency of the infarct related artery and left ventricular function as the major determinants of survival after Q wave acute myocardial infarction. *Am. J. Cardiol.*, **71**, 1–7

Murray, R. G. (1993). Which patients should have exercise testing after myocardial infarction treated by thrombolysis? *Br. Heart. J.*, **70**, 399

Stevenson, R., Ranjadayalan, K., Wilkinson, P. *et al.* (1993). Assessment of Holter ST monitoring for risk stratification in patients with acute myocardial infarction treated by thrombolysis. *Br. Heart J.*, **70**, 233–40

Stevenson, R., Umachandran, V., Ranjadayalan, K. *et al.* (1993). Reassessment of treadmill stress testing for risk stratification in patients with acute myocardial infarction treated by thrombolysis. *Br. Heart J.*, **70**, 415–20

Implantable defibrillators

Mirowski, M., Reid, P. R., Mouer, M. *et al.* (1980). Termination of malignant ventricular arrhythmias with an implanted automatic defibrillator in human beings. *N. Engl. J. Med.*, **303**, 322–4

Fogoros, R. W., Elson, J. J., Bonnet, C. A. *et al.* (1990). Efficacy of the automatic implantable cardioverter defibrillator in prolonging survival in patients with severe underlying cardiac disease. *J. Am. Coll. Cardiol.*, **16**, 381–6

Kim, S. G., Fisher, J. D. and Furman, S. (1993). Hypothetical death rates of patients with implantable defibrillators remain very hypothetical. *Am. J. Cardiol.*, **72**, 1453–5

Heart failure/prognosis

Hutchins, G. M. and Bulkley, B. H. (1978). Infarct expansion versus extension: two different complications of acute myocardial infarction. *Am. J. Cardiol.*, **41**, 1127–32

The Consensus Trial Study Group (1987). Effects of enalapril on mortality in severe congestive heart failure: results of the co-operative North Scandinavian enalapril survival study (Consensus). *N. Engl. J. Med.*, **316**, 1429–35

Pfeffer, M. A., Lamas, G. A., Vaughan, D. E. *et al.* (1988). Effect of captopril on progressive ventricular dilatation after anterior myocardial infarction. *N. Engl. J. Med.*, **319**, 80–6

The SOLVD Investigators (1991). Effect of enalapril on survival in patients with reduced left ventricular ejection fractions and congestive heart failure. *N. Engl. J. Med.*, **325**, 293–302

Pfeffer, M. A., Braunwald, E., Moye, L. A. *et al.* (1992). Effect of captopril on mortality and morbidity in patients with left ventricular dysfunction after myocardial infarction. Results of the Survival and Ventricular Enlargement (SAVE) trial. *N. Engl. J. Med.*, **327**, 669–77

The SOLVD Investigators (1992). Effect of enalapril on mortality and the development of heart failure in asymptomatic patients with reduced left ventricular ejection fractions. *N. Engl. J. Med.*, **327**, 685–91

Eng, C., Zhao, M., Factor, S. M. *et al.* (1993). Post-ischemic cardiac dilatation and remodelling: reperfusion injury of the interstitium. *Eur. Heart J.*, **14**(Suppl. A), 27–32

Cardiogenic shock

Mundth, E. D., Yurchak, P. M., Buckley, M. J. *et al.* (1970). Circulatory assistance and emergency direct coronary artery surgery for shock complicating acute myocardial infarction. *N. Engl. J. Med.*, **283**, 1382–4

Scheidt, S., Wilner, G., Mueller, M. *et al.* (1973). Intra-aortic balloon counterpulsation in cardiogenic shock: report of a co-operative clinical trial. *N. Engl. J. Med.*, **288**, 979–84

Willerson, J. T., Curry, G. C., Watson, J. T. *et al.* (1975). Intra-aortic balloon counterpulsation in patients in cardiogenic shock, medically refractory left ventricular failure and/or recurrent ventricular tachycardia. *Am. J. Med.*, **58**, 183–91

Lee, L., Bates, E. R., Pitt, B. *et al.* (1988). Percutaneous transluminal coronary angioplasty improves survival in acute myocardial infarction complicated by cardiogenic shock. *Circulation*, **78**, 1345–51

Goldberg, R. J., Gore, J. M., Alpert, J. S. *et al.* (1991). Cardiogenic shock after acute myocardial infarction. Incidence and mortality from a community-wide perspective, 1975–1988. *N. Engl. J. Med.*, **325**, 1117–22

Seydoux, C., Goy, J. J., Bevret, P. *et al.* (1992). Effectiveness of percutaneous coronary angioplasty in cardiogenic shock during acute myocardial infarction. *Am. J. Cardiol.*, **69**, 968–9

Mitral regurgitation

Wei, J. Y., Hutchins, G. M. and Bulkley, B. H. (1979). Papillary muscle rupture in fatal acute myocardial infarction. A potentially treatable form of cardiogenic shock. *Ann. Intern. Med.*, **90**, 149–53

Pinson, C. W., Cobanoglu, A., Metzdorff, M. T. *et al.* (1984). Late surgical results for ischemic mitral regurgitation. *J. Thorac. Cardiovasc. Surg.*, **88**, 663–72

Hickey, M. S. J., Smith, L. R., Muhlbaier, L. H. *et al.* (1988). Current prognosis of ischemic mitral regurgitation; implications for future management. *Circulation*, **78**(Suppl. 1), 1–51–69

Tcheng, J. E., Jackman, J. D. Jr, Nelson, C. L. *et al.* (1992). Outcome of patients sustaining acute ischemic mitral regurgitation during acute myocardial infarction. *Ann. Intern. Med.*, **117**, 18–24

Rupture of septum and free wall

Vlodaver, C., Coe, J. I. and Edwards, J. E. (1975). True and false left ventricular aneurysms: propensity for the latter to rupture. *Circulation*, **51**, 567–72

Dymond, D. S., Elliott, A. T. and Banim, S. O. (1979). Detection of a false left ventricular aneurysm by first-pass radionuclide ventriculography. *J. Nucl. Med.*, **20**, 851–4

Reddy, S. G. and Roberts, W. C. (1989). Frequency of rupture of left ventricular free wall or ventricular septum among necropsy cases of fatal acute myocardial infarction since introduction of coronary care units. *Am. J. Cardiol.*, **63**, 906–11

Lemery, R., Smith, H. C., Giuliani, E. R. *et al.* (1992). Prognosis in rupture of the ventricular septum after acute myocardial infarction and role of early surgical intervention. *Am. J. Cardiol.*, **70**, 147–51

Massel, D. R. (1993). How sound is the evidence that thrombolysis increases the risk of cardiac rupture? *Br. Heart J.*, **69**, 284–7

Oliva, P. B., Hammill, S. C. and Edwards, W. D. (1993). Cardiac rupture: a clinically predictable complication of acute myocardial infarction; report of 70 cases with clinicopathologic correlation. *J. Am. Coll. Cardiol.*, **22**, 720–6

Mural thrombus

Vaitkus, P. T. and Barnathan, E. S. (1993). Embolic potential, prevention and management of mural thrombus complicating anterior myocardial infarction. *J. Am. Coll. Cardiol.*, **22**, 1004–9

Right ventricular infarction

Cohn, J. N., Giuha, N. H., Broder, M. I. *et al.* (1974). Right ventricular infarction. Clinical and hemodynamic features. *Am. J. Cardiol.*, **33**, 209–14

Isner, J. M. and Roberts, W. C. (1980). Right ventricular infarction complicating left ventricular infarction secondary to coronary heart disease. *Am. J. Cardiol.*, **45**, 217–21

Caplin, J. L., Dymond, D. S., Flatman, W. D. *et al.* (1987). Global and regional right ventricular function after acute myocardial infarction: dependence upon site of left ventricular infarction. *Br. Heart J.*, **58**, 101–9

Creamer, J. E., Edwards, J. D. and Nightingale, P. (1991). Mechanism of shock associated with right ventricular infarction. *Br. Heart J.*, **65**, 63–7

Zehender, M., Kasper, W., Kauder, E. *et al.* (1993). Right ventricular infarction as an independent predictor of prognosis after acute inferior myocardial infarction. *N. Engl. J. Med.*, **328**, 981–8

Pericarditis and Dressler's syndrome

Davidson, C., Oliver, M. D. and Robertson, R. F. (1961). Post-myocardial infarction syndrome. *Br. Med. J.*, **ii**, 535–9

Toole, J. C. and Silverman, M. E. (1975). Pericarditis of acute myocardial infarction. *Chest*, **67**, 647–53

Cheung, P. K., Myers, M. L. and Arnold, M. D. (1991). Early constrictive pericarditis and anaemia after Dressler's syndrome and inferior wall myocardial infarction. *Br. Heart J.*, **65**, 360–2

Imaging techniques

Parkey, R. W., Bonte, F. J., Meyer, S. L. *et al.* (1974). A new method for radionuclide imaging of acute infarction in humans. *Circulation*, **50**, 540–6

Dymond, D. S., Jarritt, P. H., Britton, K. E. *et al.* (1978). Positive myocardial scintigraphy at the bedside – evaluation using a portable gamma camera. *Postgrad. Med. J.*, **54**, 641–8

Sherman, G., Litvack, F., Grundfest, W. S. *et al.* (1986). Demonstration of thrombus and complex atheroma by in-vivo angioscopy in patients with unstable angina pectoris. *N. Engl. J. Med.*, **315**, 913–19

Underwood, S. R., Rees, R. S. O., Savage, P. E. *et al.* (1986). Assessment of regional left ventricular function by magnetic resonance. *Br. Heart J.*, **56**, 334–40

Khaw, B. A., Yasuda, T., Gold, H. K. *et al.* (1987). Acute myocardial infarction imaging with Indium-111 labelled monoclonal antimyosin Fab. *J. Nucl. Med.*, **28**, 1671–8

Höher, M., Hombach, V., Hopp, H. W. *et al.* (1988). Coronary angioscopy during cardiac catheterization and cardiac surgery. *Int. J. Card. Imaging*, **3**, 153–9

Gussenhoven, W. J., Essed, C. E., Lancee, C. T. *et al.* (1989). Arterial wall characteristics determined by intravascular ultrasound imaging; an *in vitro* study. *J. Am. Coll. Cardiol.*, **14**, 947–52

Meese, R. B., Spitzer, C. E., Negro-Vilar, R. *et al.* (1990). Detection, characterization and functional assessment of reperfused Q wave acute myocardial infarction by cine magnetic resonance imaging. *Am. J. Cardiol.*, **66**, 1–9

Davies, S. W., Winterton, S. J. and Rothman, M. T. (1992). Intravascular ultrasound to assess left main stem coronary artery lesion. *Br. Heart J.*, **68**, 524–6

Holman, E.R., van Jonbergen, H.-P. W., van Dijkmann, P. R. M. *et al.* (1993). Comparison of magnetic resonance imaging studies with enzymatic indexes of myocardial necrosis for quantification of myocardial infarct size. *Am. J. Cardiol.*, **71**, 1036–40

Pennell, D. J., Keegan, J., Firmin, D. N. *et al.* (1993). Magnetic resonance imaging of coronary arteries: technique and preliminary results. *Br. Heart J.*, **70**, 315–26

Myocardial stunning, hibernation and viability

Akins, C. W., Pohost, G. M., De Sanctis, R. W. *et al.* (1980). Selection of angina-free patients with severe left ventricular dysfunction for myocardial revascularization. *Am. J. Cardiol.*, **46**, 695–700

Braunwald, E. and Kloner, R. A. (1982). The stunned myocardium: prolonged, post ischemic ventricular dysfunction. *Circulation*, **66**, 1146–9

Liu, P., Kiess, M. C., Okada, R. D. *et al.* (1985). The persistent defect on exercise thallium imaging and its fate after myocardial revascularization: does it represent scar or ischemia? *Am. Heart J.*, **110**, 996–1001

Braunwald, E. and Rutherford, J. D. (1986). Reversible ischemic left ventricular dysfunction: evidence for the 'hibernating myocardium'. *J. Am. Coll. Cardiol.*, **8**, 1467–70

Tillisch, J., Brunuw, R., Marshall, R. *et al.* (1986). Reversibility of cardiac wall motion abnormalities predicted by positron tomography. *N. Engl. J. Med.*, **314**, 884–8

Brunken, R., Schwaiger, M., McKay, M. G. *et al.* (1987). Positron emission tomography detects tissue metabolic activity in myocardial segments with persistent thallium perfusion defects. *J. Am. Coll. Cardiol.*, **10**, 557–67

Dilsizian, V., Rocco, T.P., Freedman, N. M. T. *et al.* (1990). Enhanced detection of ischemic but viable myocardium by the reinjection of thallium after stress redistribution imaging. *N. Engl. J. Med.*, **323**, 141–6

Bonow, R. O., Dilsizian, V., Cuocolo, A. *et al.* (1991). Identification of viable myocardium in patients with chronic coronary artery disease and left ventricular dysfunction. Comparison of thallium scintigraphy with reinjection and PET imaging with 18F-fluorodeoxyglucose. *Circulation*, **83**, 26–37

Tamaki, N., Ohtani, N., Yamashita, K. *et al.* (1991). Metabolic activity in the areas of new fill-in after thallium-201 reinjection: comparison with positron emission tomography using fluorine-18-deoxyglucose. *J. Nucl. Med.*, **32**, 673–8

Underwood, S. R. and Pennell, D. J. (1992). Viable myocardium and reinjection of thallium. *Br. Heart J.*, **68**, 537–9

Gropler, R. J., Geltman, E. M., Sampathkumaran, K. *et al.* (1993). Comparison of carbon-11-acetate with fluorine-18-fluoro-deoxyglucose for delineating viable myocardium by positron emission tomography. *J. Am. Coll. Cardiol.*, **22**, 1587–93

Heyndrickx, G. R., Wijns, W. and Melin, J. A. (1993). Regional wall motion abnormalities in stunned and hibernating myocardium. *Eur. Heart J.*, **14**(Suppl. A), 8–13

Rahimtoola, S. H. (1993). The hibernating myocardium in ischemia and congestive heart failure. *Eur. Heart J.*, **14** (Suppl. A), 22–6

Unusual causes of infarction

Haider, Y. S. and Roberts, W. C. (1981). Coronary artery disease in systemic lupus erythematosus. *Am. J. Med.*, **70**, 775–81

Gao, S. Z., Schroeder, J. S., Hunt, S. A. *et al.* (1989). Acute myocardial infarction in cardiac transplant patients. *Am. J. Cardiol.*, **64**, 1093–7

Mullins, P. A., Cary, N. R., Sharples, L. *et al.* (1992). Coronary occlusive disease and late graft failure after cardiac transplantation. *Br. Heart J.*, **68**, 260–5

Brecker, S. J. D., Stevenson, R. N., Roberts, R. *et al.* (1993). Acute myocardial infarction in patients with normal coronary arteries. *Br. Med. J.*, **307**, 1255–6

Index